The New Tantra
Simple & Sexy

The New Tantra
Simple & Sexy
Longer, Better Lovemaking for Everyone

Susan Crain Bakos

QUIVER

First published in the USA in 2008 by
Quiver, a member of the
Quayside Publishing Group
100 Cummings Center
Suite 406-L
Beverly, MA 01915-6101
www.quiverbooks.com

12 11 10 09 08   2 3 4 5

ISBN-13: 978-1-59233-360-8
ISBN-10: 1-59233-360-5

Library of Congress Cataloging-in-Publication Data
Bakos, Susan Crain.
  The new tantra : simple and sexy : longer, better lovemaking
for everyone / Susan Crain Bakos.
     p. cm.
  ISBN 978-1-59233-360-8
  1. Sex instruction. 2. Sex. 3. Tantrism. I. Title.
  HQ31.B23494 2008
  613.9'6--dc22
                                        2008015246

Book layout: Kathie Alexander
Photography: Jacques Seurat and Allan Penn

Printed and bound in Singapore

This book is for Carolyn Males—
dear friend, best reader, personal inspiration,
and intrepid world traveler. She is the ultimate
witty, urbane, and sophisticated woman—
and a Hot Babe—who never does anything
the way anybody's mama does.

Contents

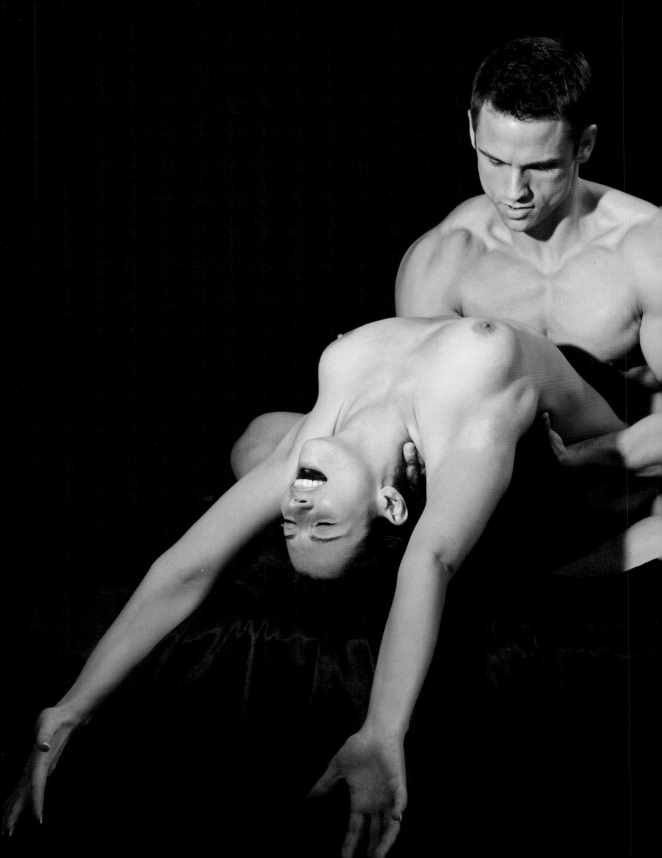

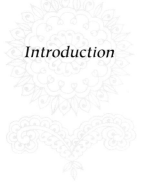

Introducing the New Tantra: Fusion Tantra

I went to hear my friend (and neuroscience researcher) Nan Wise speak as part of a sexuality panel at the New Life Expo held in Manhattan in October 2007. Her work in the neuroscience of sex is beyond interesting—it's fresh, new, and exciting! But the rest of the coma-inducing panel included a fifty-ish author/workshop leader who is still getting in touch with his feminine side; an oily, slight man whose contribution to the world of spoken sex seemed to be facilitating lame yet self-congratulatory panels; and a pretty and very thin young woman—member of One Taste, a group of "urban monks" devoted to female orgasm. These "urban monks" believe orgasm is only achieved by stroking the upper-left-hand quadrant of the clitoris. She described herself as "an orgasm messenger from God."

There were also two middle-aged women dressed as hippie gypsies who write about and teach Tantra. One of them gave the "hoo-hoo, hee-hee, haw-haw" demonstration of clearing the charkas (energy centers that correlate to nerve centers in the body) through breathing and chanting. If you didn't know she was hoo-hee-hawing Tantra (because women who dress like this have been doing that for twenty-five years), you would swear you'd stumbled into a natural childbirth class.

And that is your Mama's Tantra, an earnest endeavor undertaken by mostly white, heterosexual, middle-class, and middle-aged couples. True to their hippie-Boomer roots, many of them still smoke pot, burn incense, and believe in a fuzzy way that the powers of love and sex can take them somewhere loosely defined as "a higher plane." Tantra is the passion fix for their cozy, married sex lives. They warm to the soothing messages imparted between the silly noises— messages that could come from fortune cookies, like:

- Sex should not be goal-oriented. (It's not just about erection and orgasm.)

- There's more to sex than intercourse. (It's not just about erection.)

- Men can be passive sometimes. (It's not just about erection.)

- Tantra deepens the intimate connection between partners. (It's insurance against "cheating," the path of least resistance when erections wane.)

- Your orgasm will be diffuse and whole-bodied. (It's not just about erection or the genital response.)

And, like so many Westerners enamored of Eastern mysticism, they don't even blink at statements like "The upper-left-hand quadrant of the clitoris contains most of the nerve endings." What!? That is just not true. No research supports such a claim. And if you think some guys have trouble finding the clitoris now, imagine telling them that only the upper-left-hand quadrant of that tiny pink organ counts.

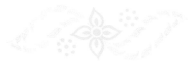

"Most of the workshops seemed a little bit silly and too woo-woo for our tastes. We didn't jive with the all-white, middle-aged, strictly heterosexual couple-oriented, New Age Tantra thing, and we ran into some trouble as we were the only queer, edgy freaky folks there."

—DR. ANNIE SPRINKLE, writing in the preface to her friend Barbara Carrellas's book *Urban Tantra*

Is This Any Place for a Hot Babe or Guy Like You?

Some teachers of Tantra and *some* couples who consider themselves serious Tantra practitioners are as smug, righteous, pompous and judgmental as *some* religious converts, vegans, members of P.E.T.A. (People for the Ethical Treatment of Animals), and others who are convinced there is only one true path and they are on it. (Our Puritan culture seems to spawn wave after wave of True Believers whose faith was based in something good and gentle before they forged it into an exclusive, self-righteous club.) "That's not Tantra" is their response to adapting Tantra techniques for use in sex that *does* put great emphasis on erections and orgasm.

Realistically, few people will practice the rigorous meditations, the chants, and chakra clearings of classical Tantra any more than they will take yoga to a comparable level or become triathletes—and that includes the Neo-Tantric practitioners who like to tell the rest of us what is and isn't Tantra. Who has the time to contemplate our navels the way the yogis did thousands of years ago? Just because most of us don't have time to throw ourselves fully into certain practices—whether it be yoga, other athletics, or even Tantra—it doesn't mean they aren't worthy pursuits for us part-time practitioners. Besides, those ancient yogis probably invented Tantra because vibrators would have been ahead of their technological time!

At first glance, Tantra might seem way behind your technological time. If you are under thirty-five, you grew up in hyperculture—which means that you live life at a rapid pace and in the "now." You're moving too fast to catch sight of the past behind you or see a clear future ahead. There is only *now*. Many of us who didn't grow up at that speed have nevertheless adapted happily to it. Whether young or not so young, most of us share a lack of patience with long processes, whether it's reading a doorstopper novel or signing on to a workout program that promises results in six months, not six weeks.

We might not be prepared to devote hours to the pursuit of bliss either, but we can use some of Tantra's basic skills as tools to make sex more focused, intense, and orgasmic.

If you have read any of my books, you know that I *do* care about my man's erection and I *do* care about orgasms, *mine*—strong, throbbing, vibrating in the clitoris, vagina, and G-spot, and sometimes radiating outward in gently crashing waves. (I can dream or think-off to those sweet little diffuse orgasms; I don't need Tantra to get me there.) Oh, yes, I care about orgasms, *his*—and yours, too. If I ran for president, it would be on a platform of "A vibrator in every nightstand and an orgasm every day." I am an unashamed and unabashed cock worshipper and I like my objects of worship big and hard. Nothing makes me feel more connected to a lover than orgasm. Or, relieves stress and tension better than orgasm. Or, for that matter, intensifies the connection I feel to my best, truest self. I come, therefore I am.

I wouldn't say that sex is *all* about erection and orgasm. (Sometimes sex is masturbation and it's all about vibes and orgasm.) But 75 percent? Maybe 80 percent? Even 85 percent? Yes, I would say that. Erection is key to heterosexual sex. Intercourse is difficult without a good erection; and for most heterosexual couples, intercourse is a big part of lovemaking. And orgasm does matter. As I've said in other books, I don't believe women when they say "intimacy" matters more than orgasm. Good sex and intimacy go hand and hand. Sex has to work—or the relationship eventually won't work either.

Yet I've been using Tantric techniques in my sex life for years. Annie Sprinkle, in fact, taught me fire-breathing. The Yabyum (sitting) position was my favorite intercourse position with a former lover, fondly recalled. I have adapted positions from the Kama Sutra for books and magazine articles. I love that first chakra, at the floor of the pelvis, the place where I do Kegels. And Tantra informed the orgasm technique I created, the Orgasm Loop.

But *my* Tantra is not your Mama's Tantra.

"The art of living Tantrically is living authentically, consciously, and sensuously. And that can be done in an infinite variety of styles and practices, all of which can bring about prolonged states of love, connection, and bliss."

—BARBARA CARRELLAS, in *Urban Tantra*

Introducing Fusion Tantra:
You Can Cut to the Chase and Still Get the Benefits

Tantra has lessons for all of us, including people like me (and probably you) who aren't going to meditate daily, even if it is physically, psychologically, and sexually beneficial. Even if you would be the one person in the room refusing to "hee-hoo-haw" if dragged to a Tantra workshop, there are lessons to be learned. In this book, we cut to the good stuff, the techniques that you can use to strengthen arousal, sustain erection, and intensify and prolong orgasm. I call this **Fusion Tantra**, because it fuses the essential skills of Tantra with everything and anything else that turns you on, from cunnilingus and fellatio to quickies—in other words, all that is often disparaged as the "goal-oriented Western lovemaking style."

I found my inspiration to write about Tantra, my way, in *Urban Tantra*, the book that Barbara Carrellas wrote because none of the existing Tantra books spoke to her, a lesbian single woman involved in BDSM (bondage and domination/sadomasochism). She and I are not on the same sex-life page and she does delve far more deeply into Tantric mental practice and philosophy than I do, but we are very much in agreement on this: There is something in the ancient way of being sexual for everyone.

Before we start, let's take a relaxing breath.

The Relaxing Breath

There's good science behind the "Take a deep breath" advice. When you take in more oxygen and regulate the rapid, shallow breathing associated with anxiety, you have let your parasympathetic nervous system (calm) take over from the sympathetic nervous system (fight-or-flight).

The relaxing breath, adapted from Tantra, both calms those jittery nerves and helps you to focus. That makes it a useful pre-seduction move as well as a good thing to do before walking into a big meeting.

You don't need to sit on the floor in a yoga position to take a deep breath. Whether sitting or standing, will your muscles to un-clench. Relax your lower belly.

Push the air out of your lungs in one long, powerful exhale. Now take a deep, slow breath that fills your lungs. Repeat, repeat, repeat.

If sex, not business, is on the agenda, clench your pubococcygeus (PC) muscle on the inhale and release on the exhale.

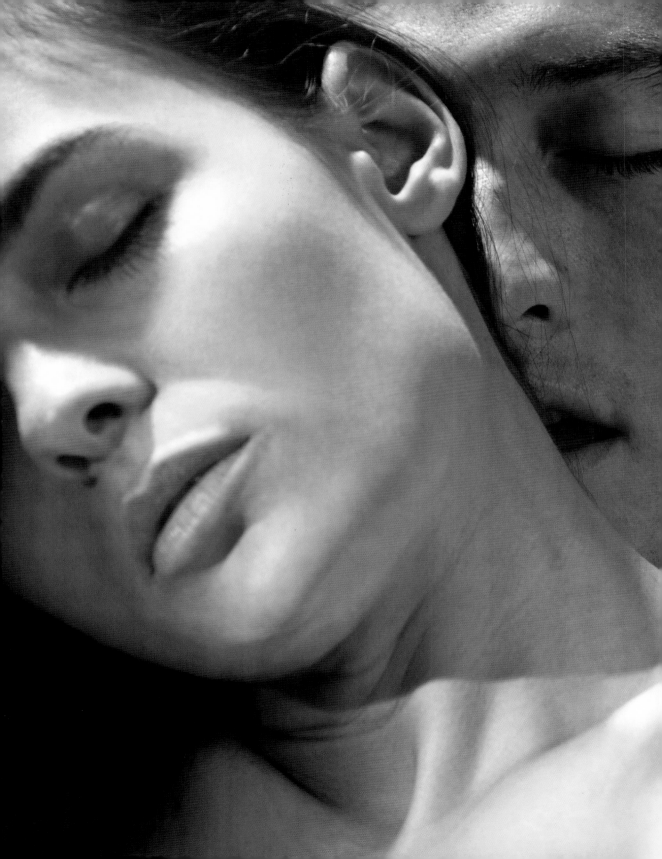

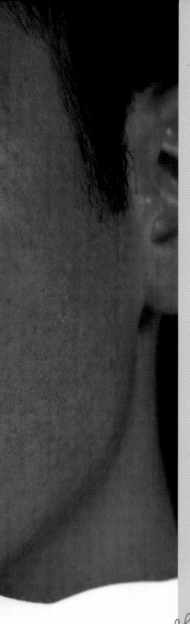

PART 1

The Bare Essentials

A Tantric devotee cornered me at a party recently in Manhattan, said she'd heard I was writing about Tantra, and wanted me to "understand" how to do it right so that I could "experience" the "intense intimate beauty of the being-to-being connection in full bloom."

I said: "You mean *orgasm*. I do and I have." Only romance novel authors use more flowery terms for sex than Tantric devotees do.

I will not speak in this spiritual jargon or call you and your lover "beings" in this book. Wordplay that obscures meaning is not essential to learning the skills that will make your sex life better. In fact, the verbiage gets in the way.

Nevertheless, before we can get into the practical aspects of Tantra in this book, some background and context are necessary. Without slipping into "woo-woo" overload here, we'll cut to just the basics. Working definitions and a bit of history are useful beginnings. We will follow in broad strokes the evolution of Tantra, the spiritual path, then we'll move through Neo-Tantra, the Westernized version, which is more about sex but heavy on the New Age "spiritual." From there, we'll progress to Fusion Tantra, which synthesizes the bare essentials into a skill set that will energize your sex life. You will see how these bare essentials are the backbone of the sexual/spiritual philosophy—yet also relevant to your twenty-first-century sex life—and discover how modern science explains the effectiveness of ancient sex techniques.

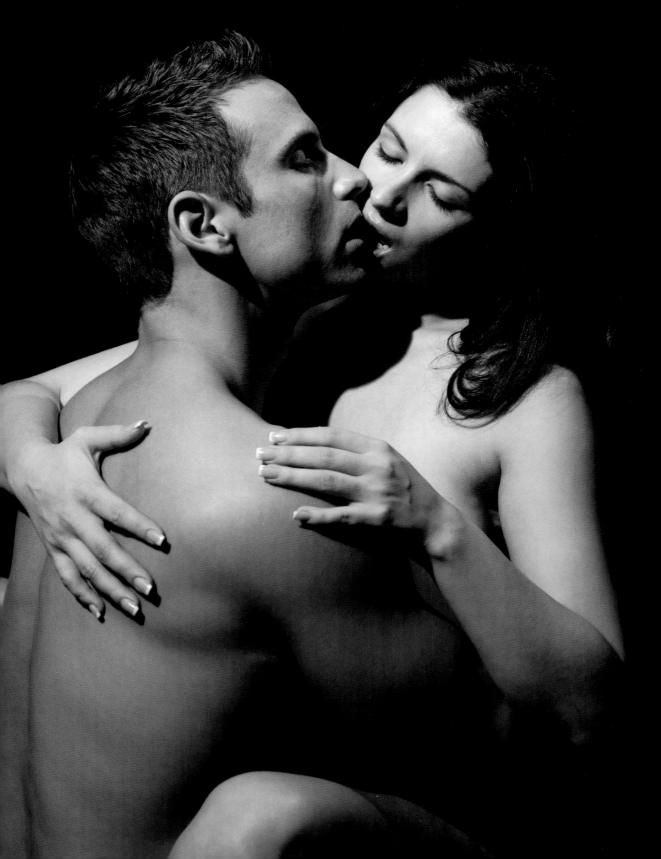

Chapter 1

Putting Tantra to Work in Your Life

Tantra is a Sanskrit word for an Eastern spiritual and sexual philosophy that emphasizes experiential approaches to life and lovemaking. The word Tantra has various translations, including "weaving," "continuous process," "manifesting or showing," and "to expand." Weaving together male (represented by the Hindu god Shiva) and female (represented by the Hindu goddess Shakti), Tantra unifies not only man and woman as lovers, but also the male and female elements within each of us.

"Tantra is an Indian philosophy that includes sexuality as a minor factor."

—SWAMI ANANDAKAPILA SARASWATI, guru/teacher

The word *being* comes up a lot in Tantra, as in "move from 'the place of doing' to 'the place of being'"—in other words, stop being so active and sit still long enough to relax inside your own skin. In commonsense terms, that can be interpreted as letting go of the tension, stress, worry, and responsibility of daily life long enough to experience desire, arousal, and release during sex with (or without) a partner. The concept of being fully conscious, or "present," in your sexual experiences is a good one.

What's with All This Talk about "Sacred Sexuality"?

Sex is sacred within Tantra, but Tantra is not "sacred sexuality," though most Western workshops and authors describe it that way. Sacred sexuality was practiced in India and other places in the Far East thousands of years ago, concurrent with the rise of Tantra. But it was the realm of temple prostitutes—courtesans reputed to commune with the gods and goddesses—not couples. Men who visited the prostitutes did learn techniques, many of which found their way into the

Kama Sutra and other sex books of the times—books written by men, for men. In those days, only men, a few wealthy women, and courtesans were literate.

We in the modern West tend to lump together the beliefs, practices, and sex techniques that have come to us from divergent sources under the umbrella of Tantra, but that is not accurate. Although Tantra, sacred sexuality, the teachings of the Kama Sutra, and other Eastern erotic arts have common points, they also differ in the same way that various Christian sects, though rooted in faith in Jesus, have their own unique beliefs and practices. It's fine to pick and choose what we want from Eastern approaches to sexuality, but it's important not to lump it all together.

We can use the main sexual lessons of Tantra in our lives. In fact, they integrate easily. Those lessons are:

- Live *in* the moment or be "present" in your sexual encounters.

- Recognize the equality of the sexes and that each of us has "male" and "female" energy.

- Extend the concept of consciousness from the mind into the body, connecting the spiritual and the physical.

- Achieve greater sexual consciousness by getting inside your sexual experience and out of your head, the place that generates all those excuses for not having sex.

- Fully connect sexually to yourself and to your partner.

- Discover your sexual energy and move it around in your body to create desire, sustain arousal, and build orgasm.

What Is Neo-Tantra?

So what about those so-called New Age Tantra devotees who criticize the rest of us for not "doing it" the right way? Well, they are wrong about Tantra, too. The sexual Tantra practiced in the West is Neo-Tantra, so named because it focuses mainly on sex, not on the classic Tantric philosophy of enlightenment. Born of religious rebellion, classic Tantra rejected the Hindu belief that celibacy was the one path to enlightenment. Yet classic Tantra, like Catholicism, has a special place in its heart for the celibate ascetic life. Those who move through and beyond passion find a kind of all-consuming, some would say "whacked out," bliss that the rest of us don't envy. Rest-assured, we are in no danger of discovering this enlightened bliss in a Neo-Tantra workshop at The Learning Annex, where the goal (whether stated or not) is to rev up your sex life in a few quick sessions.

Neo-Tantra fuses higher sexual functioning with living on a higher spiritual plane. In a typical Neo-Tantra course of study, you will activate your chakras, release your Kundalini energy, and worship the divine feminine—all to achieve whole-body orgasms. This version of super sex—a concept appealing to Westerners—is supposed to bring enlightenment with orgasm.

Nearly every Tantra teacher and workshop leader in the West is a *Neo-Tantric* practitioner. What they teach is an expansion of the minimal sexual aspects of classic Tantra (supplemented by techniques and theories from other Eastern erotic philosophies and technique guides). Then, they combine those techniques with a New Age interpretation of the spirituality lessons that can be gleaned. Though they typically claim it is, their take on the discipline is *not* pure Tantra.

Neo-Tantra versus Western Sex

According to the ancient teachers, sex in Tantra is a vehicle for spiritual transformation, the path to bliss, and a means to expand consciousness in sexual and spiritual ecstasy.

"Western sex," on the other hand, is goal-oriented, recreational, and/or mired in relationship issues. The goal of "Western sex," they say, is orgasm, not to connect or pleasure deeply.

I disagree with that. Would there be so many magazine articles and books— not to mention therapy sessions—on "intimacy" in relationships if we only cared about reaching the goal of orgasm? In fact, women aren't as orgasm goal-oriented as I wish they were. Women have too often subordinated their own sexuality to their relationships. But modern Western lovers do want it all: lusty, vigorous, orgasmic sex *and* deep, intimate relationships.

We might speak in different ways with our sexperts and Neo-Tantra teachers. The sexperts advise from this model of sex: desire, foreplay, arousal, and release. The Neo-Tantra teachers work from less concrete models, using phrases like, "only the moment with exquisite union" or "a dance with no beginning and no end" or whatever to describe sex. (What does that *really* mean, anyway?) When we cut through the vague, ethereal jargon and translate the ideas, the message of Neo-Tantra is: orgasm is nice, but it isn't essential, and you can enjoy a low state of arousal and call it "sex." That message appeals more to the older, married couples who practice it than it does to the members of xUrban Culture. But at the end of the day, we're all looking for the same thing: the most carnally satisfying and emotionally intimate sex we can get.

You and I just want to get there with enough time to spare for everything else we want to do. The basic sexual elements of Tantra can help us get there. These elements elicit the psychological, sensual, and emotional responses that intensify sex.

> *"There has always been tension in Hinduism between sexuality and celibacy. The question was: Should one be celibate or celebrate sexuality? The Hindus and Buddhists embraced Tantra and said, 'Let's have sex and call it spiritual."*
>
> —SUDHIR KAKAR, noted Indian psychologist, religious authority, and author

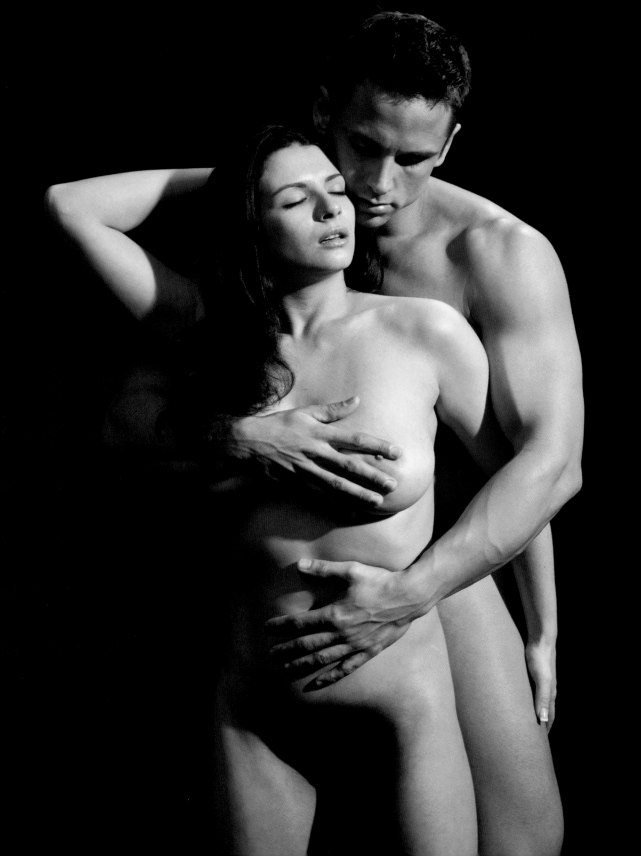

Chapter 2

Stripped-Down Tantra: The Need-to-Know Basics

The blending of yoga, meditation, and ritual that is Tantra originated in India thousands of years ago. But historians do not agree on exactly when Tantra really began, partly because it started as an oral tradition. Even the dating of early texts—and there are many of them—is up for debate. Estimates range from three to five thousand years ago, depending upon which source is cited. The Indian version of Tantra that is most familiar to us in the West began in the early centuries after the birth of Christ and was practiced by both Hindus and Buddhists.

The teachings of Tantra differed from those of Hinduism and Buddhism in a significant way: Tantra promised enlightenment through ecstasy in one lifetime. The other spiritual paths led through several lifetimes of accumulating wisdom (reincarnation) or required extreme renunciation of the pleasures of the flesh (including all but minimal clothing, food, and shelter) to reach enlightenment. (Enlightenment is a state that can probably be compared to a sense of being "one" with the universe, as our individual edges seem to blur, like melting into the cosmos.)

Tantric ecstasy did not become entirely sexual until it made its way to the West. From the beginning, Westerners confused Tantra, "sacred sexuality," and the Kama Sutra—and threw in writings on ancient Chinese sexual customs, too. For the most part, those early sex tourists just brought back the good stuff, the sexy bits.

This knowledge of Eastern sex techniques began with the Crusaders. They traveled to the East about a thousand years after Christ to spread the Gospel to the infidels, and then went back to Europe with perfumed oils and sex tricks. The nineteenth-century British explorer Sir Richard Burton was most responsible for bringing Eastern sexual philosophy and technique to the West. He translated *1001 Tales of Arabian Nights*, the Kama Sutra, *The Perfumed Garden*, and other texts. Like Dr. Alfred Kinsey a century later, Burton risked censure, ridicule, and legal action for the cause of sexual enlightenment.

In the twentieth century, techniques from the Kama Sutra were adapted in sex therapy, such as "the squeeze technique," which involves squeezing the head of the penis to delay ejaculation. In fact, Western sex therapy has focused on creating and sustaining male erection and female arousal and encouraging her orgasm—basic concepts of Eastern lovemaking arts. New Age Tantra workshops and classes sprang up in the United States and Europe in the 1970s. In the 1980s, the G-spot (once known as "the sacred spot") was "discovered."

Ancient Eastern lovemaking philosophy and technique have so informed modern theories and practices that we cannot pull the separate threads from our erotic tapestry. Fusion Tantra has been going on for some time now. I just gave it a name.

"Tantra in India in the early days probably resembled the social revolution in America in the 1960s: experimentation with sex and drugs; group ecstatic rituals with music, dancing, and sex; loving whomever you choose regardless of race or background; and questioning the moral, ethical, and philosophical precepts of the day."

—BARBARA CARRELLAS, *Urban Tantra*

Just the Basics, Please

What can we distill from these disciplines to make sex more pleasurable and in-timate relationships deeper? I took Tantra and Neo-Tantra down to the bones to answer that question. The bare essentials that follow are the concepts you need to understand and the techniques you need to learn to benefit from what Tantra has to offer.

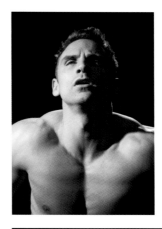

SEXUAL CONSCIOUSNESS/MEDITATION

Sexual meditation is simply meditation with an erotic focus. To practice this type of meditation, first regulate your breathing, clear your head, and mentally pic-ture an image—a flower, a vulva, a penis, an ocean view, or whatever stimulates your erotic senses. This kind of meditation is the preliminary step in focusing erotic energy. It slows down your busy mind and lets you experience the sexual energy that has been lying beneath the surface all along.

BREATH CONTROL

One of the most elegantly simple ideas in the history of the world is creating and managing erotic energy with breath. Harness your breath and use it first to focus arousal and later to increase arousal and intensify orgasm. Brilliant.

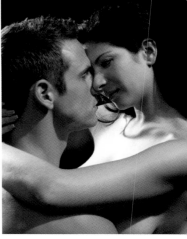

EYE CONTACT

Tantric faith holds to the maxim that the eyes are the gateway to the soul. And true Tantra practitioners spend considerable time gazing into one another's souls. They call it a new level of intimacy. Sometimes it's just TMSI (too much soul information). But making love with your eyes open (not necessarily all the time) does give it a bigger charge.

KISSING

A good kiss has always been more important to women than to men. The early practitioners of Tantra and the erotic arts knew that. The eyes may open into the soul, but the mouth takes you on the journey to somewhere else you'd like to go: the genitals.

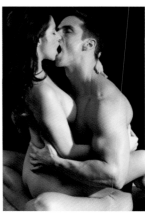

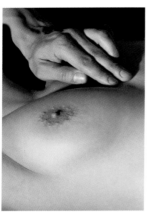

TOUCHING

Erotic touch is part of good lovemaking. In Tantra, touching is not enough. You must *become* the touch. In real terms, that means: get the pressure right. If you press too lightly or too hard, your lover either doesn't respond or pulls away. When the pressure is just right, your hand and his (or her) flesh seem to melt together. (In the overblown language of Tantra, you have *become the touch*.)

FOCUSING SEXUAL ENERGY

Sexual energy is *real* energy that you can feel and manipulate by increasing it and then moving that potent force around your body. As with the disciplines of all the martial arts, Tantra is dependent on this concept. After you have cleared your busy mind and let the erotic feelings come to the surface, you can feel the sexual energy humming throughout your body. Focusing that energy is the first step in creating strong and sustainable arousal.

MOVING SEXUAL ENERGY

The first principle of moving energy is simply this: energy follows thought. If you've never tried to move your body's energy, you might dismiss that as a conjurer's trick. It's a real thing. When you think about moving the energy, it will move.

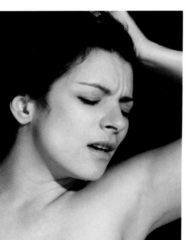

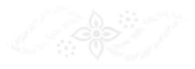

"For years, I was widely quoted on claiming that practicing Tantra enabled me to make love to my wife Trudy for up to seven hours. I was joking when I said that. The seven hours included dinner and a movie."

—STING, musician

But What About Those Seven Chakras?

I would guess there has never been a book with "Tantra" in the title and no "chakras" in the table of contents. Chakras are a significant element of Tantra, and a part of the original concept. If I don't give you the quick tour, you will feel cheated. And I can't have that.

Chakra is the Sanskrit word for "wheel," which is why the chakras are depicted as spinning spokes of energy and light. They do roughly coordinate to nerve pathways throughout the body. If you accept that energy does flow through the body, you can view the chakras as places where the energy builds and is then dispatched into other areas.

Three of the chakras are key to Fusion Tantra, but we don't have to call them by their name or make noises to clear them.

1. The first (root) chakra is located on the perineum between the anus and the genitals. You work that area when you do Kegels (see page 65) and pleasure it with G-spot stimulation or perineum massage. Let's just call this chakra by its rightful name: perineum.

2. The second chakra—the sex chakra—located in the lower abdomen below the navel, might be the most familiar because it's also called chi, the place where energy is centered in martial arts. Yoga exercises that make the pelvis more flexible and belly dancing work the second chakra—or your sexy lower belly.

3. The fourth chakra, the heart chakra, is located at the center of the chest, above the breast in a woman. Breathing exercises, especially fire-breathing, suffuse this part of the body with sexual energy. Why call it a chakra when we can simply refer to your heart and lungs?

℘ WILD CARD TECHNIQUE: **THE FIFTH CHAKRA TRICK**

Chakra number five, located at the throat, is the chakra of creative expression. Some women can reach orgasm while performing fellatio—without manual or oral clitoral stimulation—due to the sensation they experience in the throat during this act. (Really, there is a physiological connection between the throat and the vagina.) If you are one of those women, this is your extra sexual energy zone. You feel the direct connection between your mouth/throat and your genitals.

There is a quick way to find out whether you have the potential to come while giving a blow job. Suck the head of his penis and pay attention to how your throat is responding. If it seems to quiver or vibrate faintly in time with your sucking, you can do this. As you are sucking him, breathe deeply and rhythmically. Imagine that your breath is a circle of fire inhaled into your nostrils, filling your mouth and throat, and exhaled through your genitals. Flex your PC muscle in time with your breathing and sucking. It's a thrilling way to come, especially if your orgasm and his ejaculation happen simultaneously.

Is Yoga Required?

The traditions of yoga and Tantra are intertwined. Both are dependent on postures, breathing exercises, and energy control. (One branch of yoga is called Tantric Yoga.) Physical exercises in Tantra are performed in yoga poses. Breath control and meditation are important in both disciplines. So is energy focus and movement. But do you need to take a yoga class to get the benefits of Fusion Tantra? No. You will, however, pick up some yoga in the exercises you learn here, like this one for loosening your pelvis in preparation for raising the sexual (Kundalini) energy.

❧ FUSION EXERCISE: **THE ENERGY BOUNCE**

To start this move, lie on your back with your arms close to your sides, palms facing down. Then do three to five sets of this exercise:

1. Bend your knees, with your feet as close to your buttocks as is comfortable.

2. Lift your hips up and *gently* bounce your buttocks up and down, merely touching, not hitting hard against, the floor.

3. Increase the speed of your bouncing.

4. Take a break. Breathe deeply several times. Resume bouncing.

Variations: Alternate the bounce with hip circles. Swing your elevated hips to the far right and then to the far left. Now make a circle with your hips using those far points as the circumference.

What Does Fusion Tantra Leave Out—and How Is That a Plus for You?

In short, Fusion Tantra leaves out the long, boring parts of Neo-Tantra to give you a basic understanding of the most important elements for improving your sex life in a practical amount of time. (If you have the time or inclination to pursue the extended parts later, you can move on to advanced Neo-Tantra books and classes.) Most important, Fusion Tantra doesn't leave out anything that can take you higher, faster. The missing elements are:

• The rituals.

• Exercises and techniques for *extreme*, prolonged arousal and sustained intercourse.

- The New Age philosophizing on the oneness of the cosmic universe (and yada, yada, yada) that pumps up most books on the subject.

There are reasons that Tantric/Neo-Tantric sex is such a time-consuming event.

First, the sex is ritualistic. For example, lovemaking begins *every time* with the preparation of the erotic scene in careful detail. *Cosmopolitan*, *Glamour*, and other women's magazines frequently run articles encouraging women to create romantic settings for sex. That's all good. (And frankly, the magazines do it better than the Tantra guides.) But every time? I leave it to you to decide how many candles and how much incense you need to feel sexy.

Second, the goals of Neo-Tantric sex are to prolong arousal, delay intercourse and ejaculation, and generally increase the time the lovers spend in erotic contact for longer than most of us have the time or inclination to do. (And it's a key reason that Tantra traditionally appeals to midlife couples who aren't changing diapers and running soccer pools anymore, not to mention dating in the city.) Fusion Tantra prolongs and extends lovemaking in moderation, which is a more realistic goal for many of us.

Third, the more deeply you go into Neo-Tantra, the more classes and workshops you will take, books you will buy, and money you will spend—to have increasingly esoteric conversations with gurus and followers who aren't saying anything real. Fusion Tantra is designed for modern lovers—singles and couples. These people have busy, complex lives and rarely have time for lovemaking that lasts for hours. But they are interested in having better and more orgasmic sex and in feeling more intensely, intimately connected to one another. Fusion Tantra is their Tantra, an update on one of the world's oldest erotic philosophies with a greater emphasis on orgasm and oral sex.

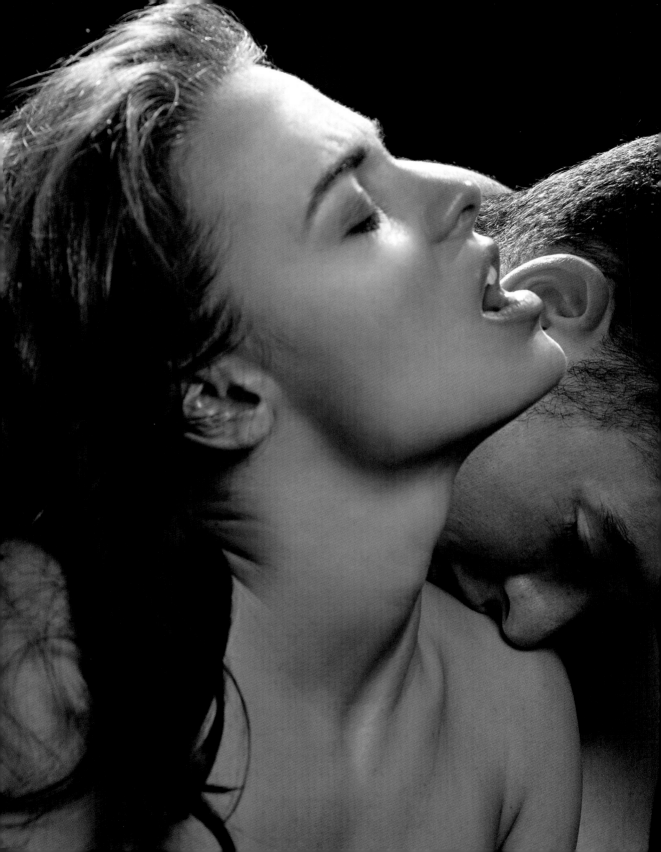

Chapter 3

Fusion Tantra's Proven Benefits

Not for nothing is Tantra sometimes called "the science of ecstasy." Much of what we know about sex in the modern age has its deep roots in early sexual teachings and rituals from the East. India really is the old country of sex. The early sexologists knew the importance of sustaining female arousal and delaying male ejaculation, and some of their techniques have been revamped and renamed as sex therapy techniques. Because they based their theories on closely observed experience, they found the clitoris and the G-spot long before Western sexologists did. They *were* research scientists.

Contrast that enlightened attitude with the prevailing primitive Western theories of sexuality based on fear, ignorance, and religious repression. A little-told story of the Crusades is the impact Eastern sexuality made on the Christian soldiers who discovered the erotic appeal of bathing and the efficacious effect that stimulating female erogenous zones had on lovemaking. Many lingered longer than absolutely necessary in the East. When they finally returned home to their dank, drafty castles in western Europe, they introduced regular bathing, the sensual delights of perfumed oils, and at least rudimentary sex techniques, a giant leap beyond yanking up her dress and entering her quickly and roughly.

No wonder the knights loomed large as romantic figures in women's fairy tales and fantasies.

How and Why Are Fusion Tantra Exercises and Techniques Effective?

There is a dearth of credible scientific research on the physical and psychological benefits of practicing Tantra/Neo-Tantra, and too much babble from self-styled gurus selling their workshops, classes, and books to seekers who don't ask the hard questions, like, "What the hell are you saying here?"

And if you look up the "science of Tantra" on the Internet, you'll also get discouraged. Here's a random example from a website article purporting to be about the science of Tantra: "In Tantra, sex is used as the cosmic union of opposites to create the polarity charge that connects with the primordial energy from which everything arises in the universe—the totality of All. We dance with the electromagnetic force field of our partner, and the dance leads to God/Cosmic Oneness."

Right.

Since vague, amorphous quotations like this one don't bring us any scientific clarity, let's instead look specifically at the individual elements of Tantra/Neo-Tantra and Fusion Tantra. The bare essentials of Fusion Tantra are the exercises and techniques with proven benefits. Exercises are activities you do—like the Kegels in chapter 9—to prepare your body for sex, while techniques provide instruction on how to perform a sexual act.

Here's what we do know in real terms about how these practices work:

- Oxygenation of the blood from breathing exercises increases circulation, which in turn increases the swelling of male and female genitals (and lubricating of the vagina).

- The combination of breathing and focusing (or meditation) reduces stress hormone levels in the brain.

- Oxygenation also boosts brain chemistry by increasing dopamine levels. (Dopamine is a "feel good" neurochemical.)

- Oxygenation enhances nerve impulses and muscle tonality as it moves down the body, making your body, including the genitals, more responsive to touch.

- Focus and breathing techniques relax the autonomic nervous system. These techniques shift control from the sympathetic (fight-or-flight) to the parasympathetic (more relaxed, reasoned) part of the system.

- Meditation regulates breathing and heart rate, reducing stress.

- Regular flexing of the PC muscles (see page 65) associated with intercourse positions adapted from the Kama Sutra increases overall sexual sensation.

The Meditation Studies

Yes, a little meditation is a good thing. Herbert Benson, M.D., a Harvard Medical School professor, published one of the first meditation studies in 1971. He found that even the most basic form of meditation produced sustained physiological benefits, such as reduced heart, metabolic, and breathing rates. His 1975 best seller, *The Relaxation Response*, inspired the nationwide growth of stress-reduction programs and clinics.

The following technique is taught widely in programs and clinics for stress reduction and relaxation.

❧ TECHNIQUE: THE RELAXATION RESPONSE

Here are the basic steps to the relaxation response (reprinted with permission from Dr. Benson):

1. Sit quietly in a comfortable position.

2. Close your eyes.

3. Relax all your muscles deeply, beginning at your feet and progressing up to your face. Keep them relaxed.

4. Breathe through your nose. Become aware of your breathing. As you breath out, say the word "one" silently to yourself. For example, breath in … out, "one," in … out, "one," etc. You can repeat any soothing, mellifluous sound, preferably with no meaning or association, to avoid stimulation of unnecessary thoughts. Breathe easily and naturally.

5. Continue for ten to twenty minutes. You may open your eyes to check the time, but do not use an alarm. When you finish, sit quietly for several minutes, at first with your eyes closed and later with your eyes open. Do not stand up for a few minutes.

6. Do not worry about whether you are successful in achieving a deep level of relaxation. Maintain a passive attitude and permit relaxation to occur at its own pace. When distracting thoughts occur, try to ignore them by not dwelling on them; just bring yourself back to repeating the word "one."

With practice, the response should come with little effort. Practice the technique once or twice daily, but not within two hours after any meal, since the digestive processes seem to interfere with the elicitation of the relaxation response.

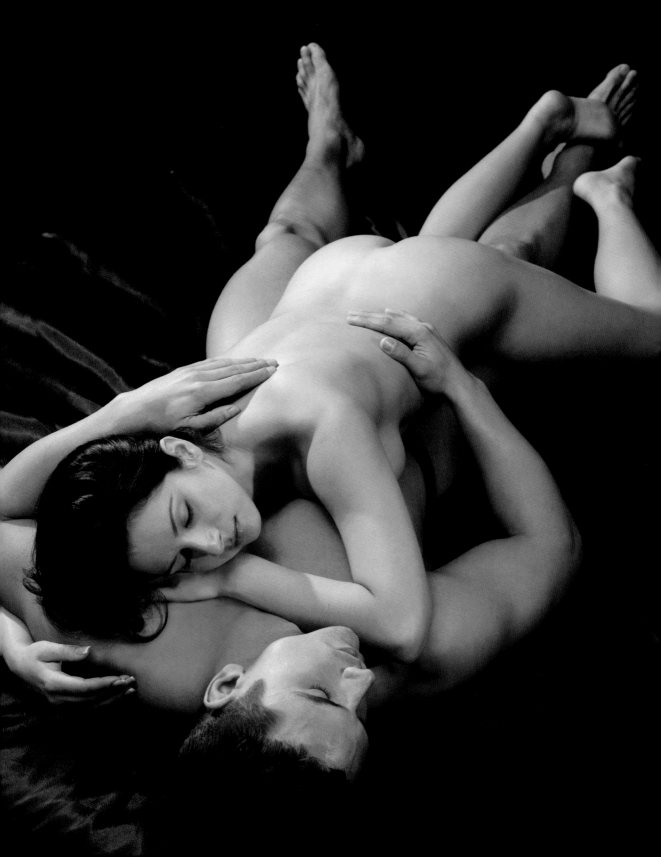

The Science of Sex: Buddhist Monks, the Dali Lama, and Your Sex Life

In September 2003, the Dali Lama, the revered Tibetan spiritual leader-in-exile, attended an Investigating the Mind conference at MIT (Massachusetts Institute of Technology), an exploration of the connections between scientific and Buddhist viewpoints on human consciousness. The Dali Lama had been meeting privately with scientists for several years, but this conference marked his "coming out" as a scientific explorer. Since then, he has taken a more public role in supporting research and encourages Buddhist monks to participate in studies on meditation.

And the monks are contributing to neuroscience research. The Buddhists have long believed that temperamental states like calmness and tranquility can be cultivated through mediation. Before advances in functional magnetic resonance imaging (fMRI) could show what was happening in the living brain, Western scientists discounted Buddhist theory. But studies conducted at Harvard Medical School, Whitehead Institute for Biomedical Research Center for Genome Research at MIT, and other places have shown that monks meditating for up to ten hours a day can change their own brain states, something previously thought impossible. They can induce compassion, for example, just by meditating on that virtue. Amazingly, their fMRI scans showed a great shift toward left frontal brain activity, which control subjects untrained in meditation could not duplicate when they were told to focus on being compassionate.

Not ready to meditate ten hours a day? Studies on the positive effects of short mediation sessions with subjects who had no meditation experience also produced impressive results. A study published in the journal *Psychosomatic Medicine* reported that subjects in a mindfulness meditation training program who meditated for fifteen minutes two or three times a week experienced emotional and immune system benefits. But what's that got to do with your sex life?

Mindful meditation with an erotic focus helps you relax your body and be more open to sexual thoughts and fantasies. Meditation also raises dopamine levels in the brain. And dopamine, of course, triggers the release of other mood-elevating brain chemicals. Erotic meditation connects that rush of good feelings with your sexuality.

The benefits of Fusion Tantra should be obvious to you now. And they can be backed up by scientific research! That's a good reason to incorporate at least some of the principles of this newly defined discipline into your sex life. It works.

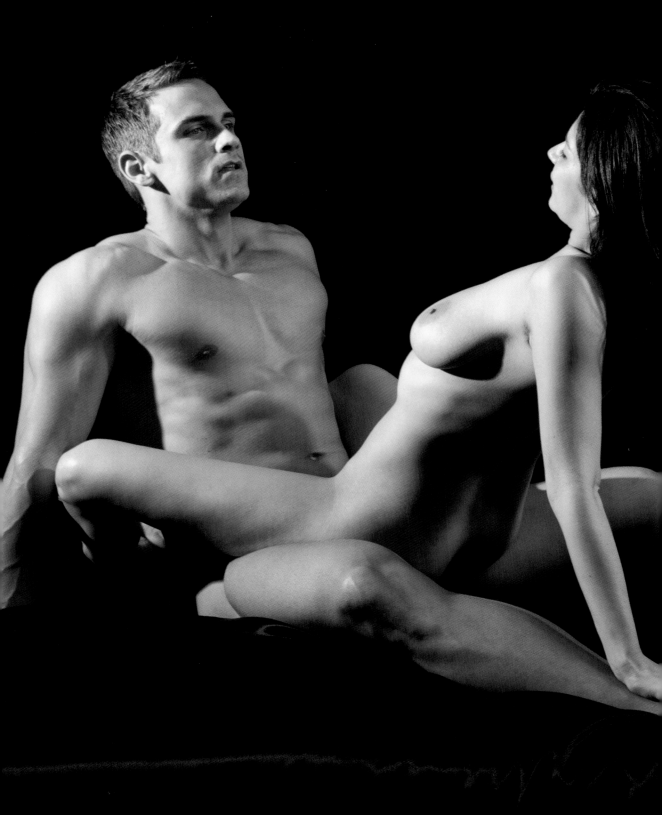

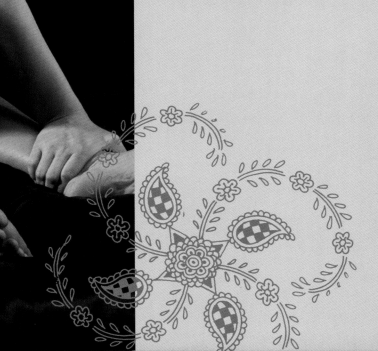

PART 2

Making Orgasm Happen —Again and Again

One of the first lessons you will learn in a Tantra or Neo-Tantra workshop is: genital orgasm is not the goal. Yet you will spend a lot of time learning how to experience whole-body orgasms. Tantra devotees seem to find the pursuit of the whole-body orgasm "purer" than going after the big genital bang.

In Fusion Tantra, we go for that big bang. The techniques are designed to bring women more quickly and easily to orgasm (and to help men delay theirs). Making orgasm a "goal" isn't a shameful thing. Women who reach orgasm easily often desire more sex and, thus, usually have more sex. Everybody is happier.

Don't even think that phrase, "I don't care if I reach orgasm or not." Yes, you do. And, yes, you will. Orgasm is one of life's worthier goals.

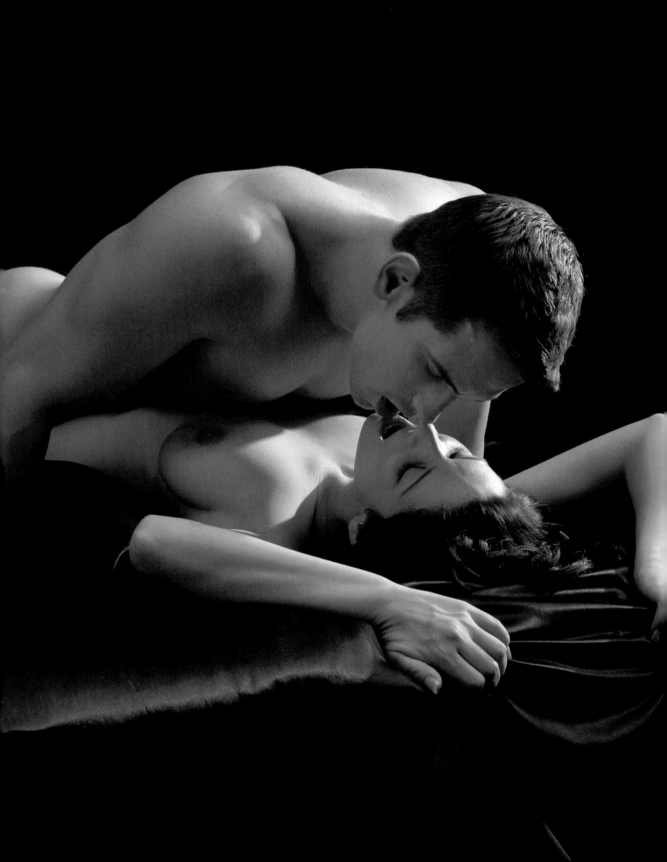

Chapter 4

The Many Types of Orgasm You Can Have

While claiming to be non-goal-oriented, Neo-Tantric practitioners seem to spend a lot of time in search of the bigger, better, stronger, longer orgasm, culminating in the whole-body orgasm. Men as well as women learn to have multiple orgasms.

If these aren't sex goals, what is a sex goal?

This is Fusion Tantra, and we don't have to claim we're in it for the cosmic bliss.

It *is* about the orgasms. The breathing techniques you've learned, combined with exceptional PC control (see page 65), energy focus, and, of course, greater sexual consciousness, will take you higher.

Why Is Orgasm So Powerful?

Orgasm is an intensely pleasurable physical and psychological response as erotic stimulation—usually genital stimulation—culminates in a release of sexual tension. The physical sensations are often more intense during masturbation than lovemaking. But having an orgasm with a partner kicks the experience up to a higher emotional level. All those feelings of closeness and affection that wash over you as the orgasmic contractions subside are triggered by the release of neurochemicals in your brain, primarily dopamine and oxytocin. It's a heady experience.

Orgasms do bring you closer together. And whether you orgasm during masturbation or lovemaking, you experience not only the release of tension but also a general feeling of well-being. Yes, orgasms make us happy.

"Every spiritual sex student really signs up for the legendary whole-body orgasm, the orgasm to get you tingling from top to toe."

—TRACY COX, sexpert and author

ORGASM IN WOMEN: THE QUICK EXPLANATION

During orgasm, the vagina, sphincter, and uterus contract simultaneously as the blood that has congested in the vaginal area suddenly rushes back into the rest of the body. The contractions generally last from three to twenty seconds, with intervals of less than a second between the first three to six contractions.

ORGASM IN MEN: THE QUICK EXPLANATION

Arousal leads to the engorgement of blood vessels in his penis just as it leads to the engorgement of her clitoris and labia. During orgasm, the blood also rushes back into his body. He experiences contractions of his penis and surrounding genital area as pleasurable sensations similar in timing, sequence, and length to her orgasm.

Why His and Her Orgasms Aren't Created Equal

A man might reach orgasm more reliably than a woman, but he doesn't have the *capacity* for orgasm that she does. Here are some of the distinctions:

- First, he doesn't have as many potential paths to orgasm as she does. He only has one (head of the penis) to her four (clitoris, G-spot, cervix, and vagus nerve, a nerve than directly connects the brain and vagina, bypassing the spinal cord).

- Second, multiple orgasms are far more likely for her because men have a refractory period—the time between erections—and women can virtually go from one orgasm into another if the stimulation continues.

- Third, extended orgasms are also more likely for her. Some women experience single orgasms lasting a minute or more and post-orgasmic contractions (sporadic erotic aftershocks in the genitals) for a minute to several minutes.

Types of Female Orgasm

There are several types of female orgasms. They include:

- *Clitoral orgasm*, which occurs primarily through stimulation of the clitoris and surrounding area.

- *Vaginal orgasm*, which occurs primarily through stimulation of the vagina (including the G-spot) and cervix via intercourse, masturbation with an internal vibrator, or manual stimulation.

- *Anal orgasm*, which occurs during oral or manual stimulation of the anus or anal intercourse.

- *Extra-genital orgasm*, which occurs through stimulation to any part of the body except the genitals, including the breasts, inner thighs, and mouth.

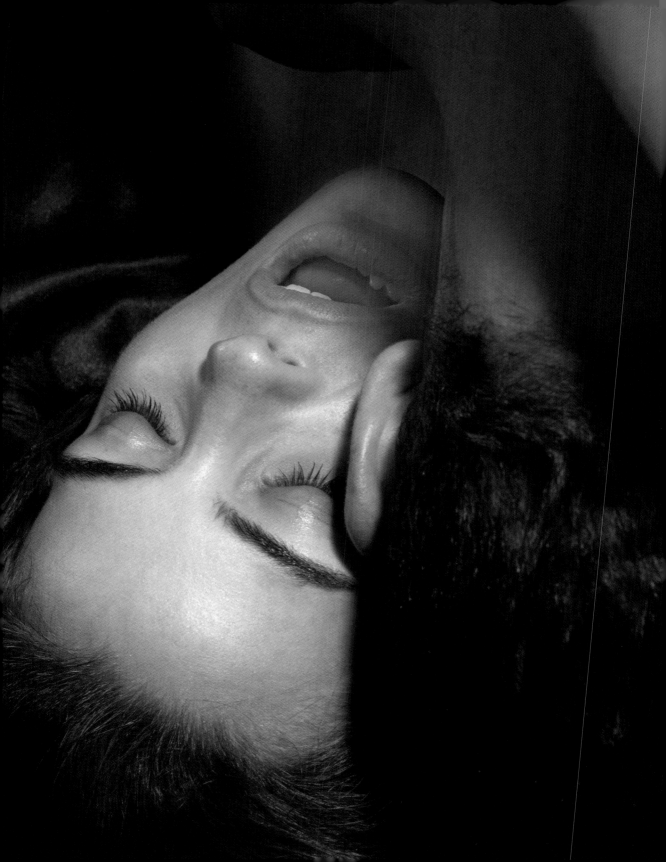

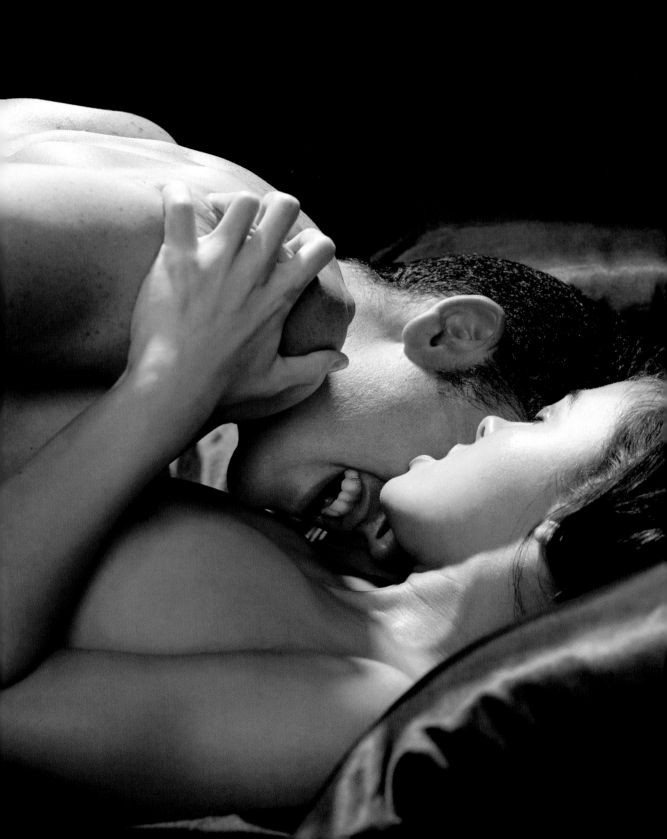

- *Blended orgasm*, which occurs through more than one form of stimulation, such as clitoral stimulation during intercourse or manual stimulation during cunnilingus.

- *Spontaneous orgasm* (also called a "no-hands" orgasm), in which women can "think themselves off" or fantasize to orgasm with no external stimulation; this type of orgasm is likely to occur while women are flexing the PC muscle. (You can also come this way using the Orgasm Loop; see chapter 6.)

There are also several types of orgasms she can have more easily and often in Fusion Tantra. These are:

- *Extended orgasms* with more contractions that last longer and might have slightly longer spaces between them.

- *Expanded orgasms* with the sensation of orgasm going beyond the genitals into the pelvic region, the buttocks, and the upper thighs.

- *Whole-body orgasms* where the sensations of orgasm are both more intense and diffuse, felt throughout the body. These are the orgasms that make you feel like the orgasm is blowing out the top of your head or shooting out your fingers and toes.

Types of Male Orgasm

The following are the two main types of orgasms men have:

- *Head of the penis friction orgasm* occurs through masturbation, oral or manual (by a partner) stimulation, and intercourse.

- *G-spot orgasm* happens through stimulation of the perineum, that little patch between the anus and the base of the testicles, or by insertion of a finger or dildo into his anus.

Men can also have different types of orgasms more easily and often in Fusion Tantra. *Multiple orgasms* are more rare in men than women because of the refractory period between ejaculatory orgasms. But some men can teach themselves to experience orgasmic contractions without ejaculation. Men can also achieve *extended orgasms*, *expanded orgasms*, and *whole-body orgasms*.

Now you have a basic primer on orgasms. Many people don't know as much about orgasms as you have learned in this chapter. In Fusion Tantra, that's just a good beginning. You'll learn even more in the next chapter, including how to have more and more orgasms. When it comes to pleasure, let's be greedy.

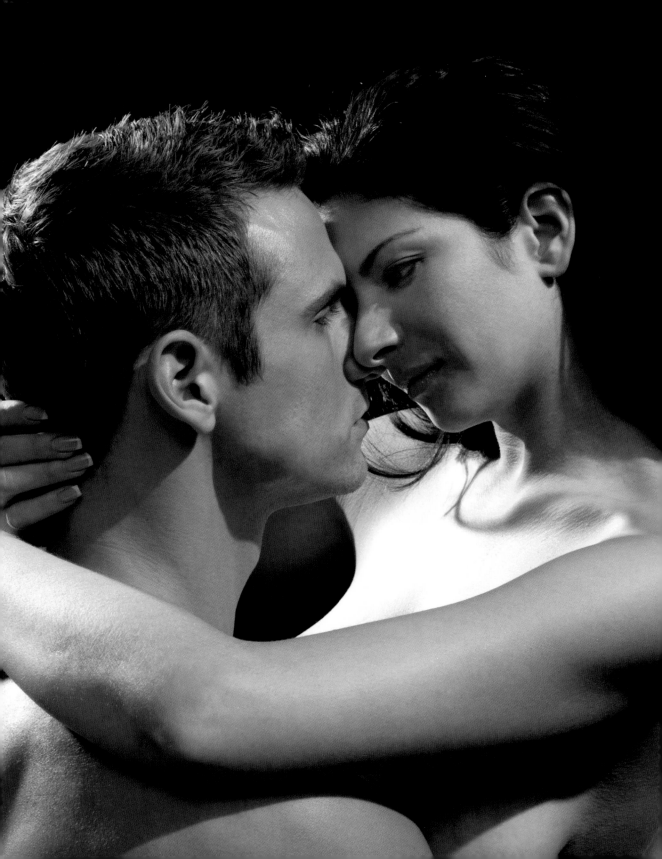

Chapter 5

His and Her Methods for Multiples

In Fusion Tantra, orgasm is a worthy goal. Yes, goal. Neo-Tantra practitioners claim that sex should be goal-free, which simply means: you might spend a lot of time touching and caressing but get no ultimate satisfaction. Not so with Fusion Tantra: intimacy through touching and caressing is great, but sexual satisfaction matters here!

Multiple Orgasms

If one is good, isn't two or more better? Yes, many of us, especially women, do feel that way. No one should feel pressured to have multiple orgasms, especially women who have difficulty achieving one. But if one comes easily, the second one is not far behind. Let it out.

HER MULTIPLES

Less than a third of women have multiple orgasms, with fewer than that experiencing them on a regular basis. Despite the numbers, it is theoretically possible for every woman who can have one orgasm to have multiples.

If a woman wants to have multiple orgasms, she can learn how to do so during intercourse, oral or manual stimulation (including the G-spot), or a combination thereof. Multiple orgasmic women typically experience more than one type of orgasm during a lovemaking session. Women who use the Orgasm Loop (see chapter 6) have a higher than average incidence of multiple orgasms—53 percent of the original 500 women in my research group had success.

There are four types of multiple orgasms: *compounded single orgasms,* in which each orgasm is distinct, separated by sufficient time so that prior arousal and tension have substantially resolved between orgasms; *sequential multiples,* in which orgasms are fairly close together, anywhere from one to ten minutes apart, and there is little interruption in sexual stimulation or level of arousal; *serial multiples*, in which orgasms are separated by seconds, with no—or barely any—interruption in stimulation or diminishment of arousal; and *blended multiples*, which are a mix of two or more of the above types.

✧ FUSION TANTRA TECHNIQUE: **BLENDED MULTIPLE ORGASMS**

Some women can only have multiple orgasms when they are receiving both clitoral and vaginal stimulation in the area of the G-spot. To achieve orgasm this way, her partner can either use his fingers to stimulate the front wall of her vagina while performing cunnilingus, or he can stimulate her clitoris during intercourse in a position that gives her G-spot stimulation.

FUSION TANTRA ORGASMS

The orgasms you have using Fusion Tantra breathing techniques, PC flexing/releasing, and energy focusing will feel different: they will be more expansive and more intense. You don't have to immerse yourself in Neo-Tantric philosophy to orgasm on a higher plane. The physical techniques take you there. They also make it more possible for you to experience multiples, expanded and extended orgasms, and that Neo-Tantric Holy Grail, the whole-body orgasm.

✧ ESSENTIAL FUSION TANTRA TECHNIQUE:
MULTIPLE ORGASMS FOR HER

Before trying this with your partner, learn how to do this during masturbation first.

1. Focus on your arousal image (see page 51). It should always be the same image and can be anything (except your lover), including a color, flowers, nature scenes, or a body part. Focus on that image until extraneous thoughts no longer intrude in your mind.

2. Breathe. Take deep, circular breaths. Imagine the circle connecting your genitals to your stomach, heart and lungs, throat and mouth.

3. Unleash your erotic energy. Feel that energy at the base of your spine and beneath your navel. Will it to infuse your genitals with heat and power.

4. Imagine your circle of breath is on fire from the energy you're releasing.

5. Begin flexing/releasing your PC muscle in time with your breathing. You might reach orgasm through energy focusing and fire-breathing alone. (But that is not a goal.)

6. Masturbate to orgasm using your fingers or a vibe.

What you do next depends on your clitoral sensitivity following orgasm:

- Sustain stimulation if you are not painfully sensitive to clitoral touch. If you continue stimulating your clitoris and surrounding genital area, and keep the breathing, PC flexing, and energy focusing going, you can come over and over again.

- Move your hand or vibrator to your vulva, vagina, or perineum, or massage your nipples or inner thighs if you are too sensitive for continued clitoral stimulation. Continue breathing, flexing, and focusing so that you remain aroused. When you are ready, stimulate your clitoris to orgasm again.

MAKING MALE MULTIPLES POSSIBLE

Men have a refractory period, a respite between ejaculatory orgasms, which varies from less than thirty minutes in young men to more than a day in older men. The refractory period limits a man's orgasm potential for multiples, unless he learns how to experience orgasm without ejaculating. Not every Western authority defines ejaculation and orgasm as separate entities in men. Some sexologists in the West are coming around to the Eastern belief that, while male orgasm typically includes ejaculation, men can learn to separate the pleasure of the rhythmic contractions from the expulsion of semen, ejaculation.

☙ ESSENTIAL FUSION TANTRA TECHNIQUE:
MULTIPLE ORGASMS FOR HIM

Learn how to do this during masturbation first before trying it with your partner. (It is more difficult to achieve than her multiple orgasms. You are not likely to learn the technique on the first attempt, so don't be discouraged.)

1. Masturbate in the way most comfortable for you, using breathing techniques to intensify arousal. For many men, that simply means working the shaft in a straightforward up and down motion.

2. Stop stroking and pump you PC muscle when you are nearing ejaculation.

3. Relax. Take deep, slow breaths. Keep working the PC.

4. Start masturbating again when arousal has subsided (but you remain erect).

5. Repeat several times, if possible.

6. Flex your PC muscle and breathe deeply while masturbating. When you feel ejaculation is imminent, continue stroking your penis while clenching your PC muscle. You should feel intense orgasmic contractions, but not ejaculate.

Nan Wise's Breathing Techniques for Spiking Any Orgasm

A neuroscience researcher and sex/relationship therapist/coach, Nan Wise is also a longtime student of yoga and former Tantra teacher. She adapted the following techniques from yoga. "These easy techniques are all about building energy and can take any orgasm higher because the energy is higher, making the release more intensely felt," she says. "And they work for women and men."

TECHNIQUE: SUSPENDED BREATH AND EXTENDED EXHALATION

As you build up to orgasm, stall your breath. Take a shallow inhale—inhale but don't "overfill" your lungs—and hold it, then let it slowly out. Keep doing this for several seconds. It should feel like you are in a place of stalled breathing because you are inhaling and exhaling small amounts of air.

Next, suspend exhalation, or, in other words, hold your breath. When you are almost at orgasm, take a deep breath. As you feel the orgasm begin, exhale in a big, extended breath while imagining sparks flying out of your penis or vagina. The exhalation should extend and expand your orgasm.

Extended and Expanded Orgasms

Extended or expanded orgasms are most likely to happen initially (or be recognized) during masturbation. You might not even notice that you're having extended orgasms with Fusion Tantra. Pay attention. Are you having more contractions that last longer and might have slightly longer spaces between them? Then you have extended your orgasms by using Fusion Tantra techniques.

If the sensations of orgasm reverberate beyond your genitals into the pelvic region, the buttocks, and upper thighs, then you are experiencing expanded orgasms.

Both extended and expanded orgasms do occur naturally after you have become proficient in the Fusion Tantra techniques of breathing, PC flexing/releasing, and energy focusing.

If you're not there yet, these two techniques can encourage extended and expanded orgasms.

❧ FUSION TANTRA TECHNIQUE: **EXPANDING HER ORGASM**

1. Masturbate using your fingers or a vibe. Once you are highly aroused, use the other hand to massage your vulva, inner thighs, and groin with light, shallow strokes. Focus on expanding the arousal in those areas as you massage them.

2. Continue massaging through your orgasm. Do you feel the orgasm in those areas of your body?

3. Count your contractions, and see whether you can have more of them the next time using the same technique.

❧ FUSION TANTRA TECHNIQUE: **EXPANDING HIS ORGASM**

1. Masturbate without ejaculating for as long as you can. Use the technique for multiple orgasms (page 45) or the basic stop/start technique, pausing whenever you feel ejaculation is imminent.

2. Let yourself ejaculate.

3. Count the contractions and notice how strong they feel. Are the first few contractions the strongest?

4. Use your other hand to massage your groin, thighs, and buttocks the next time you masturbate. Focus your arousal there.

5. Delay ejaculating for as long as possible. While you are holding back the ejaculation through PC clenching or stop/start, continue massaging. When you do ejaculate, count the contractions. Are there more? And do you feel the sensation of orgasm throughout your genitals, thighs, and buttocks?

Whole-Body Orgasms

Whole-body orgasms might take a little practice, but aren't they worth it? Often women don't have multiple or extended and expanded orgasms simply because they are in the habit of stopping with one good orgasm. Just don't stop, and see where continued play can take you. It's not as easy for men, but not impossible either. Any man who can sink a putt can surely have a whole-body orgasm.

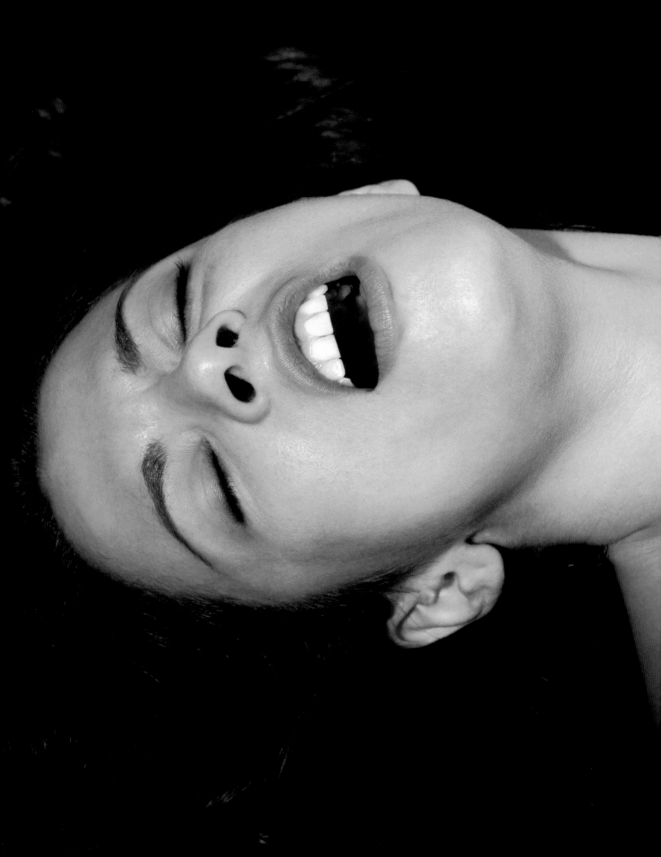

Chapter 6

How to Have No-Fail
Orgasms Everytime

In the late '80s, I took a "no-hands, spontaneous orgasm" workshop from Dr. Annie Sprinkle, famed sexologist and performance
artist. Her method of reaching orgasm without genital stimulation
was a combination of fantasy and fire-breathing. Lying on the floor
and fire-breathing with about twenty-five other women, I remember
thinking: there is a germ of a good idea here, but this is not working.

❧
Chapter Note

*You can learn everything
you need to know about
this no-fail orgasm
technique in my book,
The Orgasm Loop.
This chapter provides
you with a short-form
adaptation.*

The fire-breathing was hot, but not hot enough. I tried adding PC flexing to
fire-breathing, but that still didn't take me to orgasm without hands. It was like
inventing a new recipe. I knew it needed more—but more of what?

I read Dr. Gina Ogden's book, *Women Who Love Sex*, and thought: I want
to have what those "thinkers-off" are having. But I didn't know exactly how
they did it.

Meanwhile, the women I interviewed for books and magazine articles were
searching for a different kind of no-hands orgasm. They wanted to come during
intercourse without needing additional clitoral stimulation. In fact, the question
they most often asked me and other sex journalists, authors, and editors was:
"How can I come during intercourse?"

Other women complained that they lost erotic focus during lovemaking
because they were distracted by guilt about things they hadn't done, or concerns
about children, work, or body issues—even anger at their partners. They needed
to focus single-mindedly on sex the way men do, shutting out distractions and
giving themselves over to the sexual experience, but they didn't know how
to do that. Men do it naturally because the male erection–brain connection is
strong. A woman's genitals don't always get the sexual message to her brain, in

part because the signs of female arousal are subtler. Compounding the problem, women often have sex without fully tapping into their arousal, making orgasm problematic.

Then I read an interview with Dr. Eileen Palace, Director of the Centre for Sexual Health in New Orleans. Her research was on the sexual arousal mind/body connection—the Cognitive Physiological Feedback Loop (CPFL). Specifically, she focused on how women could learn to use biofeedback to strengthen that arousal connection.

"A man's receives cognitive feedback from his erection," she said. "Women have tingling, throbbing, and lubrication, but it's very subtle, and you can't see it. To fully enjoy sex, a woman needs something that links what's happening down below to the brain."

That was when I had one of those "Ah-ha!" moments, as I realized that women need something more practical than biofeedback. They need an arousal image, a mental focus point as powerful as an erect penis. So I had the arousal image, the fire-breathing, and the PC flexing. Yet my plan still needed something.

The Missing Piece

While visiting my sister in southern Illinois, I hooked up with Rick Hasamear, a family friend who has black belts in five different martial arts. I listened to him talk about energy focus—moving energy within the body. He can stop an arrow from being shoved into his throat using energy focus alone. (He makes his throat as hard as stone. Now that is awesome to see.) I asked him to teach me how to move my energy into my genitals and use it for erotic stimulation. He did—and then I had all the pieces of the Orgasm Loop in place at last.

Using the O Loop, Step by Step

The Orgasm Loop is designed for those women who want a no-hands orgasm during intercourse *and* those women who keep getting distracted and losing arousal. It's been tested on over five hundred women, and 85 percent of them now use it successfully. Any woman who wants a reliable means of reaching orgasm will have one using the O Loop.

The Orgasm Loop is a revolutionary technique for reaching orgasm *any time, every time, and multiple times.* It fuses cognitive feedback research on female orgasm and creative visualization therapy technique with Tantric breathing, PC flexing, *and*—a breakthrough concept—an adaptation of the same energy-focus method that allows martial arts black belts to break boards, bricks, and blocks.

The Orgasm Loop is a simple technique that any woman can master by using it several times during masturbation before taking it into partner sex. My book *The Orgasm Loop* teaches you how to use it in every sexual situation. Following are the basic directions for using the Orgasm Loop.

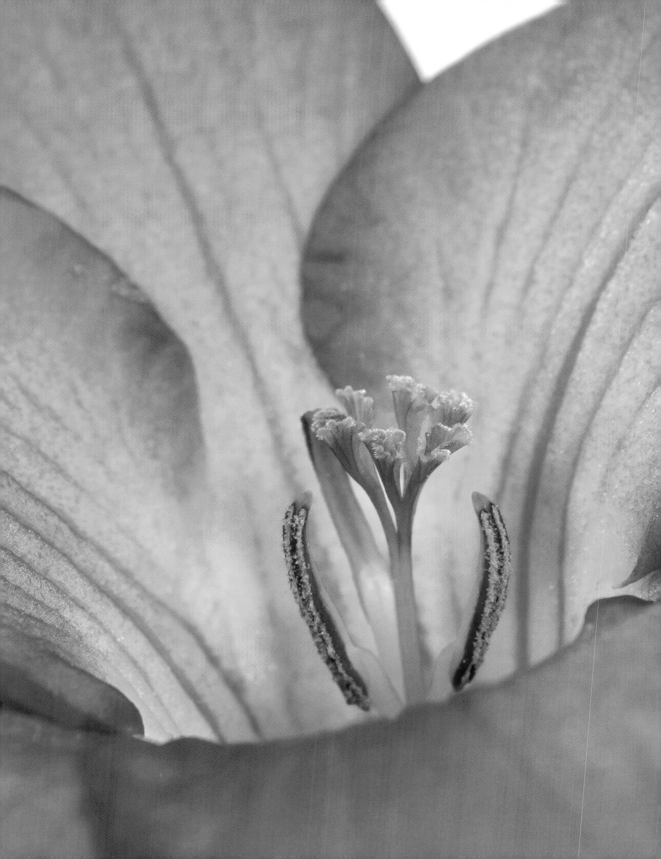

MENTAL AROUSAL

Close your eyes, clear your mind of distractions, and visualize your arousal. You need a mental picture that equates to his erection, something you see that says immediately: I am aroused. That image is a highly individual choice.

Some women might visualize their genitalia—lips swelling, moisture forming, their skin color changing to deeper pink. Other women might visualize a flower, perhaps an orchid like the one featured on the previous page. (The sensual flower paintings of Georgia O'Keefe can be an inspiration.) Some women might see arousal as a color, perhaps pink or red—or saffron yellow, the color of Devi (the mother goddess) in Hindu mythology. A beach at sunset can be an arousal image as well.

Find the image that represents arousal to you, and focus on it every time you use the Orgasm Loop. This image must become your mental erotic mantra. Focus to the extent that no other image enters your mind. (The first few times you use the Loop with your lover, keep your eyes closed during kissing and foreplay in general so you won't lose focus.)

ENERGY FOCUS

When you are conscious of nothing but arousal, turn your focus inward. Focus on a spot just below your navel (your chi). Breathe deeply and slowly, and imagine that little spot of energy glowing and growing. Move it down into your genitals with your breath.

Hold that energy in place.

Now imagine a fiery coil of sexual energy located at the base of your spine. This is Kundalini, or sexual, energy. Uncoil it and move it into your genitals. Feel the undulating, coiling energy circling around and through the spot of glowing energy.

You have moved your body's energy into your genitals, particularly the clitoris. And you are experiencing heightened sensitivity to touch now because you have created a physiological response in your body. Your heartbeat is accelerated. Your body temperature is rising. You feel more alive, more sensuous with the heat. And the blood flow concentrated in your genitals is making them incredibly sensitive.

PHYSICAL MOVES

1. While maintaining your energy focus, use breathing to intensify the mind/genital connection. Imagine you are breathing fire in a circle, inhaling it up from your genitals, throughout your body, and exhaling it out your mouth. Keep doing this in a circular fashion.

2. Once you have created a circle of fire, flex your PC muscles in time with your breathing. Tighten them as you breathe in; loosen as you breathe out. The combination of controlled breathing and energy focusing creates heat. You literally move that heat in and out of your body in an exciting circle as you fire-breathe. Like any form of deep breathing, it increases the oxygen level in the blood. And it forces more blood into your genitals.

   Keep up the fire-breathing during intercourse. Don't worry if you lose a cycle or two. Just pick it up again, especially at the point of orgasm, because it intensifies orgasm.

3. Apply clitoral stimulation, either orally or manually, or by positioning yourself in intercourse to make the connection between the shaft of the penis and the clitoris. Very little stimulation will be necessary at this point to achieve orgasm. And you can have more orgasms simply by maintaining the focus and the breathing instead of relaxing after the orgasm.

Don't be discouraged if it takes you a few or even several practice sessions to make the O Loop work smoothly for you. Some of the women in my initial test group made it work quickly. One who had never reached orgasm in any way but "marathon masturbation sessions" that left her chafed and exhausted had almost instant success with the O Loop. On the other hand, half a dozen women who "often" experienced orgasm during lovemaking before using the O Loop found that it took as many as ten sessions to "do it without stopping to think about the directions or, worse, checking the printout."

Whatever their experiences, all agreed that it was worth putting the time into the learning curve because the O Loop delivers what you need to get what you want: focused arousal and reliable orgasm.

If you are interested in learning more about the Orgasm Loop, read *The Orgasm Loop*, which teaches you how to combine the technique with other sex techniques. Kundalini energy, more fully developed in a following chapter, is another interesting topic for further exploration. Especially if you are fairly proficient in yoga already, look for a class or workshop in Kundalini yoga, which is more sexually oriented. Both the O Loop and Kundalini yoga utilize fire-breathing, which will greatly help you focus your sexual energy and enhance your overall sexual experience.

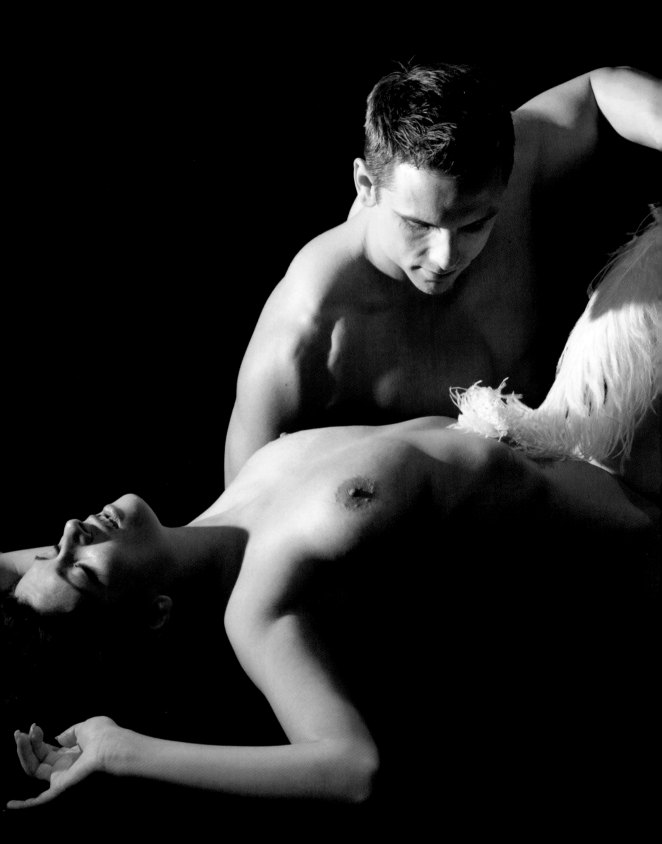

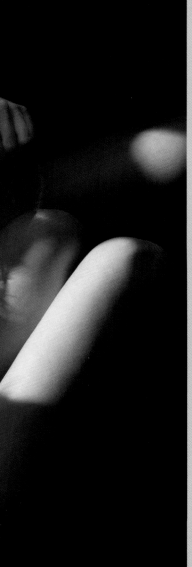

PART 3

The Essential Fusion Tantra Skills for Finding Passion and Satisfaction

The fact that you are already familiar with some, if not most, of the techniques in the Fusion Tantra bare essentials skills set just proves my point: Fusion Tantra has been underway for a long time. Western lovers have been borrowing and adapting from Eastern lovemaking arts since printed erotica has been available (even if it was under the counter). Perhaps without realizing it, most of you have used some of these techniques. You probably picked them up from magazine articles or books that seemed to have nothing to do with Tantra.

In the next sections, I'll describe many of these techniques in more detail. With each technique, I'll explain:

- What it is.

- How to do it, including, in some cases, variations that will take the technique to a higher level of performance and enjoyment.

- Why it works (the science of sexual response).

- How you can use the technique most effectively in your sex life.

The fact that I call these "essential skills" sets Fusion Tantra apart from Neo-Tantra. Neo-Tantra teachers and practitioners like to pretend it's not about the skills. Yes, it is. Good lovers are technically proficient lovers. Passion is great, but it isn't enough to take you and your partner where you want to go. How many women fall asleep dissatisfied after lovemaking because neither their passionate lovers nor they had the skills to bring them to orgasm? We'll have none of that "passion without satisfaction" in Fusion Tantra. Read on, and learn the skills that will blend both together for you.

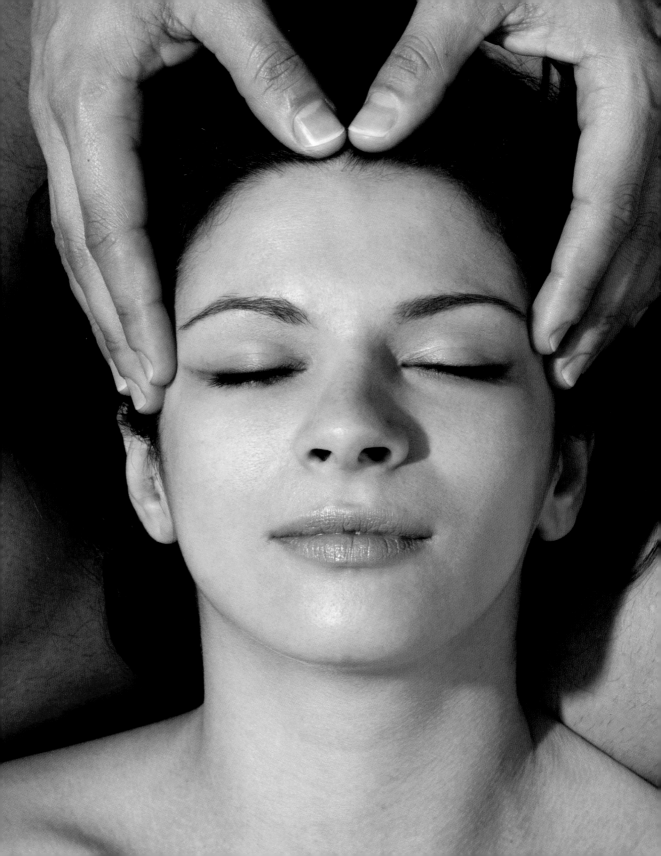

Chapter 7

Set the Scene for Passion: Develop Your Sexual Meditation and Breathing Skills

Sexual meditation is simply focusing your thoughts on erotic images that stimulate you. The connection between meditation and raising your libido is fairly obvious. (As you think, so you are.) But why do breathing techniques have the same effect? They increase oxygenation, which stimulates arousal—and they make us feel sexier because a change in breathing reminds us of arousal.

Staying Fully in the Present

If you've tried the basic relaxation exercise on page 31, you have already discovered that meditating is nothing more than sitting down in a quiet place and emptying the clutter from your mind.

Although the steps to practicing meditation are simple, the results can be complex. According to Margot Anand, author and perhaps the premier Tantra teacher in the world, "everything comes up" in sexual meditation. It brings out all your timidity and fear, anxiety and reluctance to let go in sex and in love.

One of the goals of Tantra is to be more mindful during sex, meaning we want our minds to be filled with the sexual moment, not our fears and anxieties that are rooted in past sexual encounters.

Sexual meditation will leave you in the present, so you can be intensely aware of your sexual sensations and, ultimately, enjoy sex to the fullest.

> *"Most of the problems people have with sex come down to this: They are stuck in their heads, not in the moment. When you get out of your head, you can be counted present in your sex life."*
>
> —NAN WISE, sex and relationship coach and creator of The Desire Curve

❧ ESSENTIAL FUSION TANTRA EXERCISE: **SEXUAL MEDITATION**

Set aside ten to fifteen minutes, preferably three times a week, to practice this exercise. Even if you only have time to try this once a week, you'll still reap the benefits.

1. Wearing loose and comfortable clothing, sit or lie down in any position that feels right to you.

2. Take long, slow, deep breaths. Clear your mind.

3. Focus on an image that will become your arousal image. It can be a color, flower, scene from nature, body part—anything but your lover. If you are mad or sad at your lover, you will focus on those feelings and not on your own arousal. Even if you're happy with him (or her), you can't make your arousal dependent on that feeling.

    Keep your focus on that image. Continue breathing in a pattern of long, slow, deep breaths.

4. Relax. See where you arousal image and your breathing take you.

Sexual meditation is extremely important. Women especially don't give themselves permission to think/fantasize/meditate on sexual imagery disconnected from their lover. But when we do, we reinforce our own sexuality—our desires and responses—apart from our lovers. We begin to own our sexuality.

Tap into Your Arousal with Breath Control

I cannot overstate the power of breath in Fusion Tantra. Breathing relaxes and focuses you. It helps create and sustain arousal, and it intensifies orgasm.

Aligning your breathing with your partner's puts you in limbic attunement, meaning your respiratory systems are on the same track. That can make you feel more intensely connected and increase the feelings of intimacy. Breath control is the first essential skill you need to acquire as you work toward achieving this.

❧ ESSENTIAL FUSION TANTRA EXERCISE: **THE CIRCLE OF BREATHING**

Breathing in a circle gets your energy moving. You can sit, stand, or lie down to do this exercise.

The circle of breath can be as big or as small as you'd like. At first, keep the circle tight—your breath should cycle through your nose, mouth, throat, heart, and lungs. As you do this, you are using energy to shake off fatigue and reinvigorate your body and mind. Once you feel comfortable, expand the circle. Allow your breath to cycle through your nose, mouth, throat, heart, lungs, and then belly and genitals. When you do this, you are creating erotic energy. Following are some step-by-step pointers for practicing this exercise:

1. Breathe gently through your nose. Feel the breath in your throat. You can also open your mouth slightly and breathe through your nose and mouth at the same time. (Try it both ways and see which one you prefer.)

2. Imagine the inhalation going from the back of your throat into your heart and lungs (and further down). Let each exhalation fall into the next inhalation.

3. Feel your breathing as a continuous smooth circle. Once you feel your breath as a circle, simply make the circle bigger.

❧ ESSENTIAL FUSION TANTRA EXERCISE: **THE BREATH OF FIRE**

The Breath of Fire is the quickest way I know to jump-start either my energy or my libido. It oxygenates the blood quickly, truly building your fire. The exercise is simple: take rapid, rhythmic, and shallow breaths through your nose while keeping your mouth closed. Breathe this way for one to three minutes.

❧ ESSENTIAL FUSION TANTRA EXERCISE: **FIRE-BREATHING**

Adapted from Kundalini (sexual) yoga, fire-breathing is a powerful tool for creating and expanding erotic energy. It is a key element in my Orgasm Loop technique. You will be surprised at how easy fire-breathing is to learn and how much it adds to your sex life. Here are the steps to fire-breathing:

1. Lying on your back, knees bent, feet spaced well apart, bring your breath deeply into your body. Imagine that the huge intake of air goes all the way into your genitals. Pull your belly button in as you exhale, pushing the air out of your body.

2. Begin panting after a dozen or so deep breaths by breathing rapidly from your belly with your mouth open. Do this ten or twenty times, then breathe deeply, inhaling through your nose and exhaling through your mouth. Make the breathing a continuous circular motion.

3. Now, imagine a circle of fire, beginning as a small circle composed at first of only your nose and mouth. Then expand the circle to include your chest and belly, and finally to include your genitals. You should feel the erotic heat moving throughout your body in a circle as you breathe.

Personal Foreplay

Erotic meditation and breathing are like the foreplay you give yourself. When you practice erotic meditation, you'll feel as aroused, if not more aroused, as after the initial kissing, caressing, and stroking that you have previously defined as "foreplay." Now just wait until we step up the foreplay, too, in chapter 11.

"The only time we ever think about breathing is when we have trouble doing it, yet conscious breathing can be a powerful aid in sexual growth."

—MARTY KLEIN, Ph.D., sex therapist

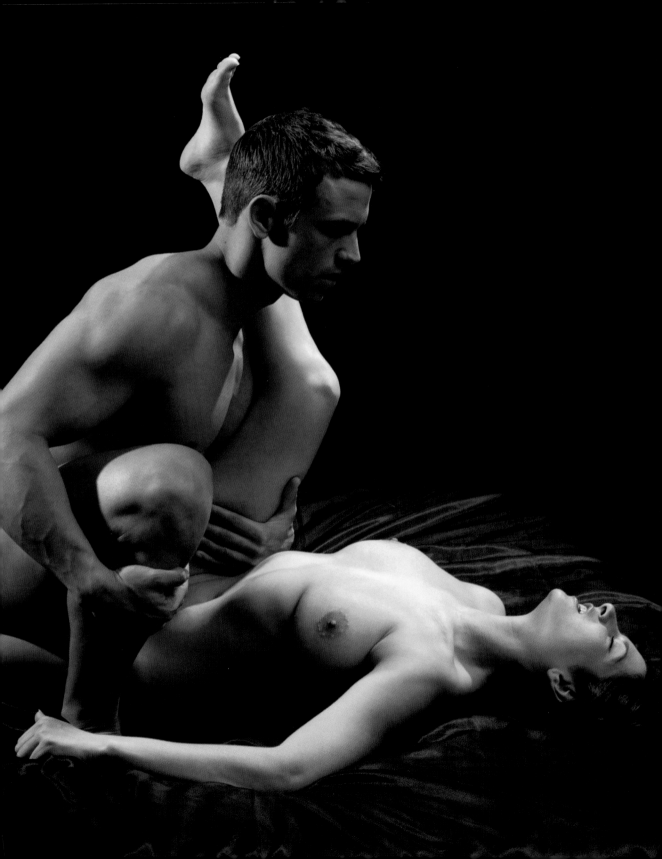

Chapter 8

Ways to Awaken Your Sexual Energy

Picture energy flowing throughout your body in the same way that blood does. In its pure form, Tantra is based on the belief that energy flows through the chakras (energy centers) from the genitals through the spine, stomach, throat, and forehead, and to the top of the head, the place of enlightenment. Energy flow really is as critical to Tantra as blood flow is to the life of the human body.

✂ FUSION TANTRA EXERCISE: **FEEL YOUR SEXUAL ENERGY**

Before you can move sexual energy around, you have to feel it. This technique is based on a rudimentary exercise taught in martial arts courses for "proving" that energy exists in the body.

1. Rub your hands together rapidly and vigorously as if you were scrubbing dirt off. Rub for ten to fifteen seconds. Stop. Hold your hands, palms facing, an inch apart. Do you feel a hot magnetic field coursing between your palms?

2. Rub your hands together in the same way again for another ten to fifteen seconds. Stop.

3. Repeat the process. Do you feel the energy more strongly now?

4. Cup one hand over your genitals and will the energy from your palm into that part of your body. Can you feel that sexual energy now? If you can't, repeat the exercise over the next few days until you can.

Kundalini: Intense Sexual Energy

In the disciplines of yoga and Tantra, sexual energy is considered intensified life energy and called Kundalini. You might have seen drawings of Kundalini energy represented as a snake coiled at the base of the spine. To further complicate things, Kundalini yoga is a separate yogic practice and, in the West, it has a stronger sexual orientation than the prevailing Hatha yoga. (In the East, Kundalini yoga is a more rigorous path toward enlightenment that is meant to take devotees to ecstasy "beyond sex.") If you have experience with martial arts, you know this Kundalini energy as "chi," or the life-force energy.

☙ FUSION TANTRA EXERCISE: AWAKENING YOUR KUNDALINI ENERGY

You can do this alone or with your partner. If you do it together, stand facing one another. Close your eyes if you like.

1. Standing, take a slow, deep breath and exhale it just as deeply. Pull the breath down and out through the seat of the Kundalini at the base of your spine, instead of collapsing the breath in your chest and lungs or stomach. Repeat the breaths and imagine that you are moving more deeply into the seat of your Kundalini with each exhalation.

2. Now raise your head as you inhale and lower your head as you exhale. Imagine you are uncoiling the energy snake and raising it up with each breath. Feel the energy flowing throughout your body.

☙ FUSION TANTRA EXERCISE: RAISING YOUR KUNDALINI ENERGY

Bring your Kundalini energy higher. Again, you can do this alone or with your partner. If you do it together, face each other and hold hands loosely.

1. Bounce gently on the balls of your feet, then slowly squat down to the floor.

2. Rock gently back and forth while resting on the balls of your feet. Feel the Kundalini energy uncoiling inside you, it's power rising. Stand up slowly.

3. Repeat the squatting and standing in a rhythmic pattern until you feel your Kundalini unfurled and coursing powerfully through your body.

☙ FUSION TANTRA EXERCISE: CONNECTING KUNDALINI ENERGIES

This is definitely a couple's exercise.

1. With knees slightly bent, stand facing one another. Make sure you are close enough to touch easily.

2. Gaze into one another's eyes. Regulate your breathing so that you are inhaling and exhaling at the same time. Open your arms wide and hold them around one another's bodies without touching. Can you feel your own energy and your partner's energy radiating between your bodies? Now put your arms around one another's shoulders loosely.

3. Breathe together and concentrate on moving your energies back and forth between your bodies. Can you feel the sexual energy pulsating through your bodies? With a little practice, you will.

❧ FUSION TANTRA EXERCISE: **ENERGY-FOCUSING AWARENESS**

You feel that energy. Now put it to work in your body. Use it to make sex hotter than it has ever been.

1. Close your eyes. Pick one finger and focus your mind solely on it. Imagine you are sending your breath to this finger instead of exhaling it out of your nostrils. (Do you feel your finger filling with warm breath?)

2. Visualize light—from the sun, moon and stars, or a bright lamp—shining down on that finger. Focus your mind on your finger, breathing and bathed in light.

3. Feel your pulse beating inside it. That finger is suffused with energy. Run it along your throat and neck, up and down your arm, across your pulse. Do you feel the energy? If not, repeat the exercise. Keep trying whenever you have a few minutes. Soon, you will feel it.

Moving and Owning Sexual Energy

Now that you feel the sexual energy, moving it within your body is simple. Energy follows thought. And it follows sexual stimulation. Sexual energy goes where you want it to go and creates intense erotic sensations. Control that energy and take your sex life to a higher level.

❧ FUSION TANTRA EXERCISE: **PULLING THE ENERGY UP**

1. Begin on your hands and knees. Inhale, sucking in your stomach as you do. Exhale, releasing your stomach.

2. As you inhale, imagine a small fiery ball of sexual energy just below your navel. Suck in your stomach. Will the energy to move through and out of your body as you exhale. Inhale, pulling the energy back into your body.

3. Repeat for a few minutes. Each time you inhale, the energy builds. When you stand up, your body will be suffused with sexual energy.

> *"When Kundalini energy is aroused by sexual activity via the root chakra, it travels up through and energizes all the chakras, revitalizing body and spirit."*
>
> —ANNE HOOPER, British sexologist and author

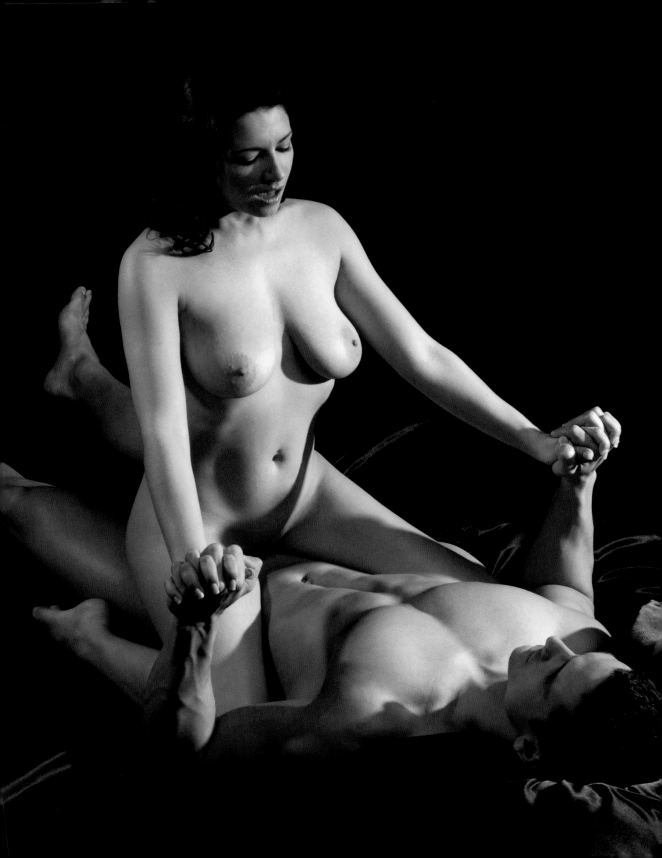

Chapter 9

Use Your Secret Weapon: PC Muscle Control

Many of the sexual positions I've selected as the essentials (following in part 5) require a strong pubococcygeus (PC) muscle, so let's tackle that before we go there. You won't derive the full Tantra benefits (such as sustaining and intensifying arousal and improving orgasm) without the ability to flex your PC muscle strongly and rhythmically. Even positions that don't strictly require strong musculature will be more pleasurable for both you and your lover if you are in great pelvic-floor shape. Yes, *both*. Men have PC muscles, too, and they need to work them out just as women do. Fortunately, the workout is basic and easy.

Kegel exercises to strengthen the PC muscle are essential for every woman and man who wants good sex. Why?

- A strong PC muscle makes orgasm more likely for women and more intense for both men and women.

- It facilitates multiple or extended orgasms in women and in some men.

- A woman with a strong PC will have some control of thrusting and depth of penetration during intercourse *and* she will be able to do some amazing tricks simply by squeezing and relaxing her PC muscle around the shaft of his penis.

- Regular Kegels keep the vagina toned after childbirth, and even after menopause.

Her Kegels

Kegels are particularly important for women. The exercises are integral for pregnant women who are getting ready for delivery and aiming to stay in shape after the baby is born. All those Kegels ensure that women who have had children won't be peeing their pants in later years. The importance of Kegels for maintaining good sex in general, but especially after childbirth, can't be understated!

Before you can do the strengthening exercises, you first have to locate and feel the PC muscle. After you've done that, the exercises should come easily.

✤ ESSENTIAL FUSION TANTRA EXERCISE: **BUILDING PC POWER**

The PC muscle is a hammock-like muscle that stretches from the pubic bone to the coccyx (tailbone) and forms the floor of your pelvic cavity. Locate your PC by stopping and starting the flow of urine. Once you have located the muscle, begin with:

- *A short Kegel sequence.* Contract the muscle twenty times at approximately one squeeze per second. Exhale gently as you tighten only the muscles around your genitals (which includes the anus), not the muscles in your buttocks. Don't bear down when you release. Simply let go. Do two sets twice a day. Gradually build up to two sets of seventy-five per day.

- Then add: *A long Kegel sequence.* Hold the muscle contraction for a count of three. Relax between contractions. Work up to holding for ten seconds, and relaxing for ten seconds. Again, start with two sets of twenty each and build up to two sets of seventy-five. You will be doing three hundred repetitions a day of the combined short and long sequences.

- Then add: *The push-out.* After relaxing the contraction, push down and out gently, as if you were having a bowel movement with your PC muscle. Repeat gently. No bearing down.

Now create Kegel sequences that combine long and short sequences with push-outs. After a month of daily repetitions of three hundred, you should have a well-developed PC muscle. You can keep it that way simply by doing one set of 150 several times a week.

Since Kegels are key to your sex life, however, you don't want to get bored with the routine and stop doing them. Shake it up with these variations.

❧ FUSION TANTRA EXERCISE: **THE KEGEL LEG CROSS**

1. Lie on your back, legs straight. Do a Kegel and hold the contraction as you pull in your stomach.

2. Raise your right leg while still holding the contraction, to form a right angle to your body. Open your leg wide to the right, return to center, cross the leg to the left of your body. Release the contraction.

3. Repeat using your other leg. Do three sets of ten with each leg.

❧ FUSION TANTRA TECHNIQUE:

HEIGHTENING ORGASM WITH A PC SQUEEZE

I adapted this technique from *The Good Girl's Guide to Bad Girl Sex* by Dr. Barbara Keesling, one of my favorite sister sexperts.

1. Caress your genitals to arouse yourself.

2. Insert your finger into your vagina when your genitals are swollen and lubricated. Tighten and relax your PC muscle around your finger. Do this repeatedly.

3. Stimulate your clitoris and fire-breathe—inhale and exhale deeply, imagining your breath is a circular track of fire coming in through your nose and going out through your vagina and back again.

4. Intercept your orgasm as you feel it approaching by doing a PC squeeze.

5. Now squeeze your PC as hard as you can and see how dramatically that affects your orgasm.

His Kegels

First, guys need to locate this muscle. As in women, the PC muscle is a hammock-like muscle that stretches from the pubic bone to the coccyx (tailbone) and forms the floor of your pelvic cavity. Locate your PC by stopping and starting the flow of urine. You can also insert a well-lubricated finger into your anus and feel the PC contract around it.

Once you have located the muscle, begin exercising it regularly, every day for a month and then at least three times a week after that. These four sets of male Kegels all produce the same effects if you do them regularly. By strengthening the musculature, you improve circulation and nerve functioning. Master each set and then mix them up.

Fusion Tantra Tip:
The Kegel Crunch

Vary your Kegel routine by doing them while exercising. For example, do Kegels as you perform pelvic crunches. Contract your PC as you pull in your stomach muscles. Release both at the same time.

❧ ESSENTIAL FUSION TANTRA EXERCISE: **QUICK CLENCHES**

1. Clench and release you PC quickly in ten-second patterns, holding the clench for ten seconds and holding the pause for ten seconds. Do three sets, and then take a thirty-second break.

2. Clench and release for five seconds with five-second pauses; repeat this ten times.

3. Clench your PC and hold for thirty seconds, then release for thirty seconds; repeat three times.

❧ ESSENTIAL FUSION TANTRA EXERCISE: **THE LONG BUILD-UP**

- Squeeze your PC and hold for a count of five. Release. Without a pause, repeat ten times.

- Squeeze and release in long and short intervals for counts of ten. Repeat three times.

- Now squeeze your PC and hold it as long as you can. The goal: two minutes. Work your way up to that.

❧ ESSENTIAL FUSION TANTRA EXERCISE: **THE RAPID SQUEEZE**

Squeeze (as tightly as you can) and release your PC repeatedly, beginning with a set of thirty and building to a hundred.

❧ ESSENTIAL FUSION TANTRA EXERCISE: **THE EASY SQUEEZE**

Squeeze and release your PC in any pattern for at least two minutes a day. Gradually work your way up to two hundred flexes.

❧ WILD CARD TECHNIQUE: **PC PLAY FOR TWO**

This takes a bit of cooperation, but if you can't cooperate while intimately connected, when can you? (And it's worth it. I promise.)

1. While you're having intercourse in any position, stop moving, but don't withdraw your penis. Ask her to be still.

2. Squeeze and release your PC. This might feel like you're tapping her G-spot.

3. Let her squeeze and release her PC now. If her muscle is very strong, she will be able to move your penis in and out by squeezing and releasing alone.

4. Sustain PC play until you just can't stop yourself from thrusting or she can't stop herself.

❧

Essential Fusion Tantra Tip: The Wave

This is a popular move in both yoga and Tantra classes taught in Hawaii. Use it to loosen up and practice your Kegels.

1. Stand with feet apart, roughly in line with your hips, knees slightly bent.

2. Imagine you are surfing a wave. Swing your pelvis forward—in the way that surfers do on the board—with the rest of your body following that pelvic lead. Arch your back at the top of your imaginary wave. Now swing back as the wave dips.

3. Once you have the movement, add Kegels.

4. Contract at the top of the wave, and release in the dip.

The Secret Weapon

I have been telling women (and later also men) to do their Kegels since I started researching and writing about sex more than two decades ago. No one single thing you do will have a more direct positive impact on your sex life. A strong PC muscle speeds arousal, intensifies orgasm, and allows you to give your partner more pleasure, too. All that for exercises that take only minutes a day. How can you not do them?

What Five Men Say About ... Kegels

"I started experiencing better erections a few weeks into doing regular Kegel sets."

—ALAN, 38

"Erections weren't an issue for me, but controlling them was. I can keep myself from ejaculating by pulling up, or squeezing in, the PC. That helps me last maybe two minutes longer, but two minutes is long in intercourse time."

—SEAN, 29

"If I squeeze and release the PC during the buildup to orgasm, I can prolong that high arousal phase a little—and get a really strong orgasm."

—BRIAN, 34

"I'm a little embarrassed to say this but—wow!—I shoot farther now. I am sure that male porn stars are working their PC muscles like crazy to get those cum shots. Now I know their secret."

—TODD, 30

"When my girlfriend gave me the directions for Kegels, I thought it was girly stuff, but I gave it a try. I've been doing Kegels for over a year and I can hang a washcloth over my erections. The sex is better, definitely better, because I have more control."

—JAMES, 37

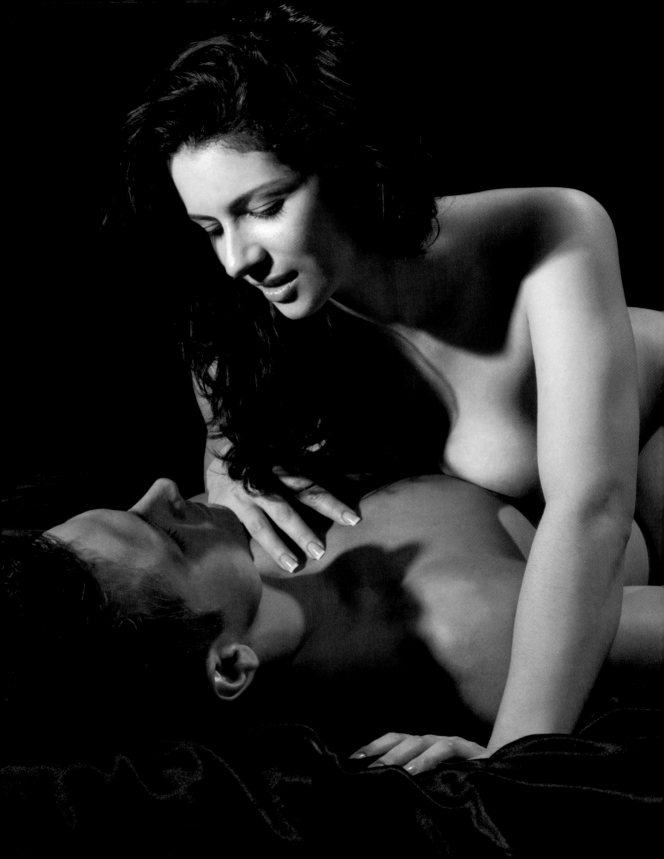

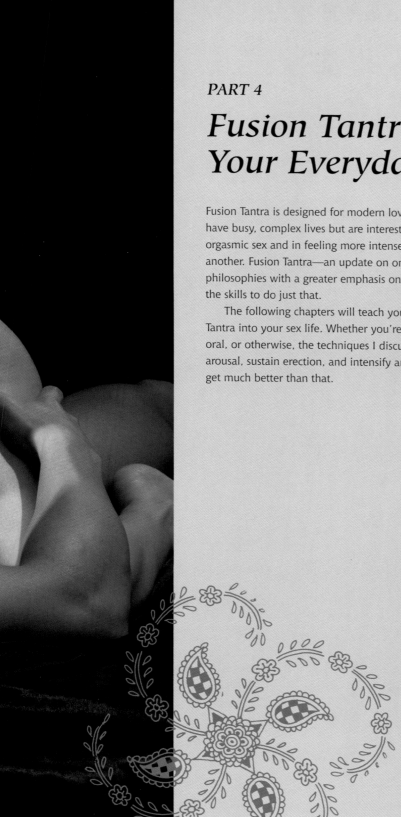

PART 4

Fusion Tantra Meets Your Everyday Sex Life

Fusion Tantra is designed for modern lovers—singles and couples—who have busy, complex lives but are interested in having better and more orgasmic sex and in feeling more intensely, intimately connected to one another. Fusion Tantra—an update on one of the world's oldest erotic philosophies with a greater emphasis on orgasm and oral sex—provides the skills to do just that.

The following chapters will teach you how to incorporate Fusion Tantra into your sex life. Whether you're engaged in solo sex, foreplay, oral, or otherwise, the techniques I discuss can be used to strengthen arousal, sustain erection, and intensify and prolong orgasm. It doesn't get much better than that.

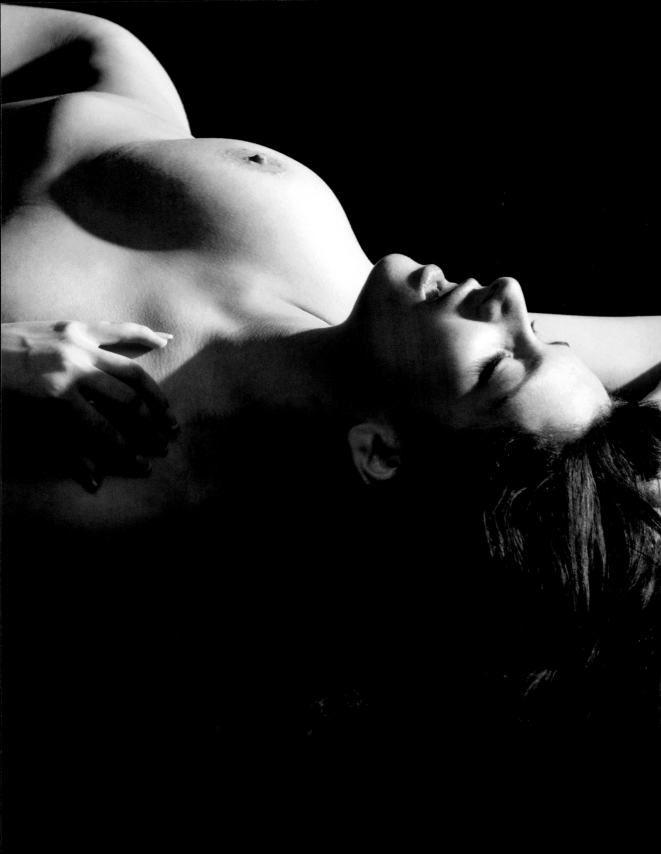

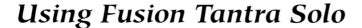

Chapter 10

Using Fusion Tantra Solo

Y ou don't have to be married (or in a relationship) to put Fusion
Tantra to good work in your sex life. And if you have a partner
who says, "I don't want to do that," you can do it without him or
her. Unlike Neo-Tantra, which is all about couples, Fusion Tantra is
about *you*.

Fusion Tantra Masturbation

Many people only know themselves sexually within the context of a relationship.
They might masturbate hurriedly for release, or not at all, out of guilt, mistakenly
believing that masturbation is "cheating" on their partner. The beauty of exploring your sexuality alone is that you gain not only a better understanding of what
turns you on but also a deeper sense of who you really are.

   Whether you're in a relationship or alone, it's a good idea to masturbate often.

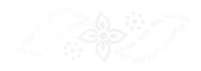

*"In Tantra, we recognize the self as the Beloved. And, YES,
recognizing yourself as your Beloved can definitely help
you attract a partner."*

—LAURIE HANDLER, Tantra teacher and author

❧ ESSENTIAL FUSION TANTRA TECHNIQUE: **MASTURBATION**

Masturbation is an essential sexual skill, whether or not you are utilizing Fusion Tantra techniques. Women learn how to reach orgasm during masturbation. Men can learn how to prolong arousal and delay orgasm during masturbation. Yet in Tantra and Neo-Tantra, masturbation is given short shrift because the focus is on the couple's lovemaking. In Fusion Tantra, masturbation is essential because it is the place where you can perfect fire-breathing and PC flexing without the distraction of a partner.

1. Start in a comfortable position, and take long, slow, deep breaths for a minute or two.

2. Focus on your arousal image.

3. Once your mind is clear and focused, begin circular breathing.

4. Stroke and fondle your genitals.

5. Combine breathing and PC flexing.

6. Now move your sexual energy into your genitals.

7. Add fire to your circle of breath.

8. Stimulate your genitals in whatever way pleases you (including with a vibe) while fire-breathing and PC flexing.

9. Use your PC muscle to intensify contractions as you near orgasm.

❧ FUSION TANTRA TECHNIQUE: **THE SOLO EYE LOCK**

Here is a new twist on open-eyed sex. Masturbate in front of a mirror. As you come, make deep, intense eye contact with yourself. (And if you want to whisper something like, "You're a sexy, Babe," that's good, too.)

Why? Loving yourself with open eyes is a big confidence boost. This technique will help you become more comfortable in your own skin. You've probably never looked into your eyes when you've come. And you'll be surprised at the beautiful woman or man you discover in there. You'll see that you look—and, hopefully, feel—sexual, sensual, and powerful.

A Quick Way to "Enroll" Your Partner in the Program

What if your lover says, "No, thanks, no Fusion Tantra for me"? That's okay. You can do the exercises and learn the techniques and put them to use, even if your partner isn't supportive. Once he (or she) sees the benefits of Fusion Tantra for you, he might change his mind. (Have you noticed that women more often do the reading and research and teach men the new tricks? The truth is that women, not men, often take the initiative in expanding our sexual repertoire as a couple.)

If you want to pull him or her into it to a small degree, here are some tips:

- Synchronize your breathing with his (or hers) as you are lying together in bed.

- While kissing, deliberately inhale his exhalation and exhale your inhalation into his mouth.

By doing these things, you lover will be a little bit in sync, whether he realizes it or not. The beauty of Fusion Tantra is that its celebration of The One is not limited to this section of the book. Many of us have sex but are not in committed monogamous relationships. Aren't we entitled to the benefits of Fusion Tantra, even during occasional trysts with a sex buddy, married lover, or friend with benefits, as well as during masturbation? Yes, of course we are! In fact, most women and men will be without a regular partner for some period of time in their sex lives. And most women and men will not feel emotionally connected to their partners all the time. The good news is the sex can be great anyway.

Enjoy yourself.

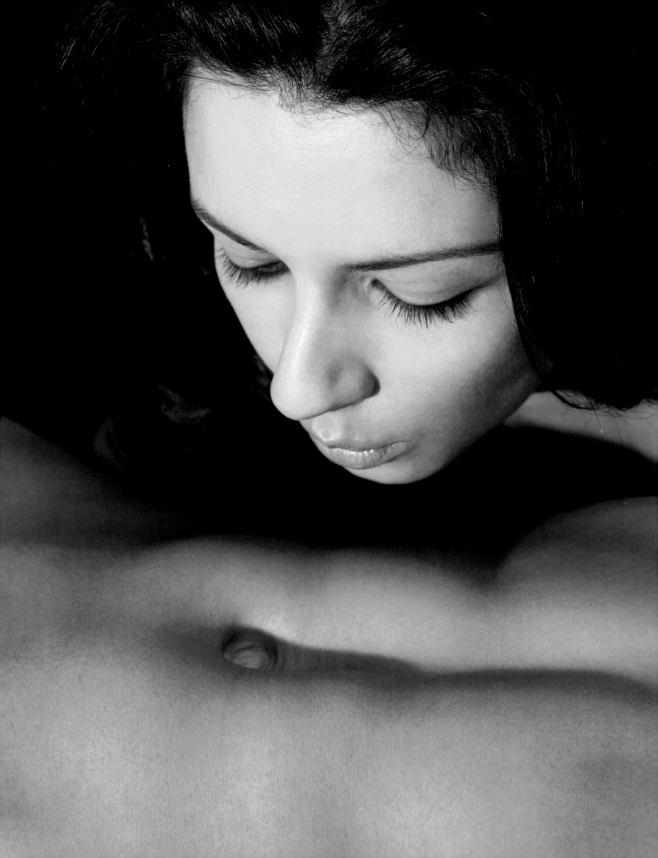

Chapter 11

Learn the Right Touch: Bringing Fusion Tantra into Foreplay

Fusion Tantra foreplay isn't like your mama's foreplay, partly because you have already aroused yourself through erotic meditation. You're starting on warm. That allows you to move more quickly and easily into higher arousal states with techniques that are aimed at both the body and the emotions.

Deepen Your Connection with Eye Contact

Making love with your eyes open is an indispensable element of Tantra/ Neo-Tantra. Eyes-wide-open lovemaking has also become a "must do" of Western sex technique. You see lovers gazing raptly into one another's eyes at the moment of orgasm in mainstream and porn films. Closed eyes, like dark bedrooms, are associated with shyness or repressed sexuality. In fact, open eyes is so damned politically correct now that you might want to close yours in defiance.

And sometimes that's a good thing. You don't always have to connect with your lover through your eyes. Maybe you just want to float on a sea of darkness, linked to the other only by touch. Or maybe you are angry with your lover. It's easier to have good angry sex if you don't have to look too closely at one another.

Often, however, you will want to keep your eyes open. Eye contact during lovemaking does deepen intimacy. Looking into your lover's eyes can make you feel more naked than being physically naked.

As you are kissing, caressing, and touching during foreplay, occasionally make deep eye contact with one another. Hold the look. Each time you do this, you will feel more strongly connected, as if your eyes exerted some magnetic pull on your lover's soul.

Maintaining eye contact at the point of your orgasm, especially if he or she is not coming simultaneously—and, really, how often does that happen?—is even more intense. Has your partner ever whispered, "Give me your orgasm"? Keep your eyes open and you have given the orgasm and more.

Spark Your Sexual Chemistry: The Kiss

The kiss is that place where we test our sexual chemistry with another person. Sexual chemistry is really a chemical reaction as we exchange biological signals with our saliva. The sensitive nerve endings on the lips, tongue, and elsewhere inside the mouth react quickly to delicate erotic stimulation from the tip of another tongue. The olfactory nerve cells in the nose are near the mouth. We really do taste, touch, and smell each other in a deep kiss. A good kiss is a good start.

❧ FUSION TANTRA TECHNIQUE: **THE SOUL KISS**

Lustier than the Sex Kiss that follows, the Soul Kiss is an improved version of French kissing.

1. Lead with the tip of your tongue in playing with your partner's lips, tongue, and the inside of his (or her) mouth. Never intrude your full tongue into his (or her) mouth.

2. Pull back before your lover can engage you in tongue wrestling.

3. Circle your lover's tongue with the tip of yours again and again—and keep pulling back.

4. Thrust the tip of your tongue in and out in a rhythmic, stabbing movement once you are both very aroused. Your lips are passionately locked, but your tongues are not fighting over the territory.

5. Tease one another only with the tips of those fast-moving tongues.

6. Don't let your hands be idle while you're kissing. Run your hands up and down one another's bodies. Let your caressing and stroking heat up as the kisses do.

7. Pull back from the deep French kiss and use the tip of your tongue in circles just inside your partner's lips.

8. Tease those lips again and again with the circling tip of your tongue, the way you tease the head of his penis in the silken swirl (this is simply just swirling your tongue around the head of his penis as you hold it in your mouth).

9. Stop.

10. Suck your partner's lips gently, one at a time.

ESSENTIAL FUSION TANTRA TECHNIQUE: **THE SEX KISS**

In Neo-Tantra workshops, the Kiss is an exercise in sharing breath, typically demonstrated with her sitting on his lap. The couple press their foreheads together, play with each other's lips, and inhale and exhale into one another's mouths. (Bring your own breath mints.)

This is nice, but I knew it could be hotter. The Sex Kiss is neither as down and dirty as the Soul Kiss, nor is it a soft and sweet expression of love between soul mates. It says: *I want you NOW, but I'm in no hurry.*

When you do this, you should be facing one another, but she doesn't have to be sitting on his lap. Whether the lovers are sitting, standing, or lying down, the one who initiates the kiss takes the other's face in her/his hands. For simplicity's sake, let's assume he is the initiator this time. Here's how it works:

1. Cradle her face in your hands while holding her gaze.

2. Start the kiss gently by licking the edges of her lips with your tongue and then lightly sucking each lip before pressing your closed mouth fully against hers.

3. Your partner responds by licking and sucking your lips and returning the closed-mouth pressed kiss.

4. Your eyes remain open as you kiss with more intensity, mouths opening gradually, the tips of your tongues engaging one another and exploring lips and tongues.

5. Pull back, kiss her neck and the tops of her breasts as she massages your shoulders, touches your chest, and runs her fingers through your hair.

6. You both explore one another's mouths with lips and tongue.

7. You pull apart when you are both aroused by the kissing.

8. You bring your lips back together in a loose, open-mouthed kiss (no tongues), exchanging your breath. For example, you exhale into her mouth as she inhales and vice versa. You gaze into one another's eyes as you breathe, kissing with more passion.

Intimacy Progresses: Touch

Like kissing, touch is basic to good sex. One of the first decisions we make about a prospective lover is whether or not to let him (or her) touch us beyond the initial hand on the arm or shoulder. When another's touch feels right, we relax. More intimate touches follow. Soon enough, we crave that touch.

In Fusion Tantra, touch is highly refined, but learning how to touch in this sophisticated way is not complicated. Tantric jargon can be off-putting. The directive to "become the touch" is a good example.

What does "become the touch" mean? It's about touching your lover with such exquisite attention to his (or her) response that you exert exactly the right pressure at the right time. In other words, pay attention to your lover's arousal level, and you will know if he wants a lighter or firmer touch. Getting the touch right is part instinct, part the result of the chemistry between you and your lover. When the chemistry is right, it makes the touch "feel right." But the largest part of "becoming the touch" simply involves paying close attention to your lover's response.

Touch is a varied repertoire to serve a varied palate. What feels good when you are really hot—like pinches, squeezes, and bites to the nipple—would likely feel harsh as an initial touch.

❧ FUSION TANTRA EXERCISE: HEAD-TO-TOE TOUCH

There are some basic touching strokes that are sensuous and arousing on any part of the body. As you are lying in bed together or cuddled on the sofa, try them on each other's head and scalp, face and neck, chest/breasts, stomach, thighs, or genitals. Vary the intensity of pressure according to your lover's response and mood.

Do you feel your lover's skin growing warmer beneath your touch? Does your lover's breathing pattern change? Do you sense that s/he leans into your touch? These are all ways of gauging responsiveness. Following are some ideas to make the most of sensuous-touch opportunities:

- *Probing fingers:* Rest you hand with fingers loosely open on part of your lover's body. Use your thumb and forefinger to lightly stroke and massage her skin. Occasionally squeeze gently with your full hand.

- *Mini massage:* Using your fingertips only, give him a tiny massage on a small part of his body, such as his thigh or arm. Let your strokes vary from walking your fingertips along his body to pressing in gently and rotating your fingertips in a circular fashion.

- *Knuckle massage:* Use your knuckles to massage her skin lightly. This is especially effective on the scalp but also feels like a new and different (and creative) touch on other parts of the body.

- *Long strokes:* Run you fingertips in long strokes across his skin. This is very effective on the forehead, neck, and chest.

- *Press stroke:* If you have ever gently and repeatedly pressed your own temples to ease stress, you know how good the press stroke can feel. Try it on your lover.

- *Pulse hold:* Lightly encircle your lover's wrist with your hand. Put a finger on her pulse and hold it there until you feel her pulse as part of your skin.

Go for the Happy Ending

Do you want to give him a happy ending? If all this kissing and caressing has given him a major erection, you might want to release the pressure for him (and for your later benefit, too).

❧ FUSION TANTRA TECHNIQUE: **THE RELIEVING HAND JOB**

1. Straddle his erection, but don't insert it inside you. Lower your breasts to his body and tease his nipples by rubbing yours across his.

2. Move down his body and kneel between his legs.

3. Take his testicles between your fingers and gently thumb them, one at a time. Hold a testicle in the palm of your hand and tickle it lightly with the pads of your fingers. Now do the same with the other one.

4. Hold the base of his penis in one hand and work your other hand in a circular fashion to the head. Use the palm of that hand to caress the head.

5. Start at the base and place your palms on either side of his penis. Use a rolling/rubbing motion—as if you were building a fire with his penis as the stick—to massage him.

6. Roll/rub in a corkscrew motion up to the head and back down to the base, keeping his penis between your palms. Start slowly. Increase speed and pressure as he gets close to orgasm.

7. Lean forward so that he ejaculates onto your breasts.

Foreplay As Its Own Play

In Fusion Tantra, foreplay is more than the fast track to intercourse (or oral sex) and orgasm. The techniques are designed to heighten arousal. You will feel the pleasure of kissing, touching, stroking, and caressing more intensely. And you'll enjoy the path to your erotic destination more than ever.

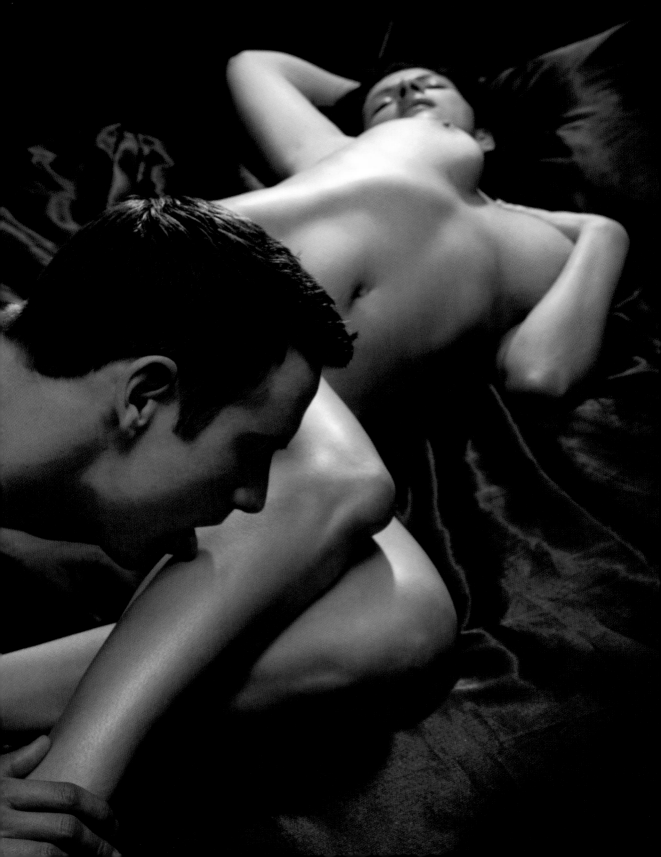

Chapter 12

Turn Up the Heat: Oral Sex, Fusion Tantra–Style

You probably think that the teachings of Tantra and the Kama Sutra place great emphasis on oral sex. And why wouldn't you? The *yoni* and *lingam*, symbols of female and male sexuality, were objects of worship in ancient India especially, but also in China, Japan, Egypt, and Greece. More to the point, Neo-Tantra, in embracing sacred sexuality, emphasizes oral lovemaking skills. But let's go back to the original sources. The teachings of Tantra and the Kama Sutra seldom refer to oral sex. The Kama Sutra, in particular, equated "sex" with intercourse. The belief in the power of the penis was pervasive. Many positions were designed to make a small penis "feel big." There's not much room for the tongue in penis-centered sex.

The Kama Sutra details eight ways a eunuch can perform fellatio, but they are not imaginative moves. In reading the Kama Sutra and other writings from that time, I concluded that a "blow job" was almost a medicinal experience— something men needed occasionally for release when there was no time or opportunity for intercourse with a woman. The eunuch was only a serviceable mouth brought in to get the job done. Refinement of technique wasn't required.

Cunnilingus is not explored at all in the Kama Sutra. And why would it be? Men believed in the power of the penis to drive their women wild with desire. It probably never occurred to them that women might also like a quick oral orgasm every now and then. And who would perform that unmanly act?

Oral sex (as fellatio) was practiced by eunuchs—and eunuchs lost their genitals in the first place, so they could be trusted with the harem women. The masters were not likely to send in the tongues.

Surely there were women in the harem who found oral pleasure with one another (and probably with a brave or reckless eunuch, too). But they couldn't read or write, so how could they share their techniques with the world? And would they have likely risked the wrath of their powerful lovers even if they could?

Modern lovers, male and female, need to be skilled in the oral arts. Fusion Tantra reflects my faith in the power of the orgasm and expertly performed oral sex. Men today know that they can reliably give a woman an orgasm via cunnilingus. And women know that nothing else compares to the thrill of power and control they feel when they hold a penis in their mouths. I have long contended that for a woman to be judged a great lover she needs to have only two skills:

1. Reaching orgasm herself, easily and often.

2. Performing the perfect blow job.

Fellatio in Eight Moves

My first thought upon going to the source, the fellatio instructions in the Kama Sutra, was: you call *that* a blow job?

I've kept the number of moves in the basic Kama Sutra directions for fellatio, and I've summarized the instructions in the first lines. But in my version of this essential Fusion Tantra technique, I've added more interesting and varied strokes. You've got a penis in your mouth. And you want to have some fun with it.

Get into a comfortable position, either kneeling at his side on the bed, at a right angle to his body, or between his legs. Or you can bring him down to the edge of the bed and kneel on the floor.

1. Warm his flesh.

When the master called a eunuch to help with his bath, he often had something more in mind. The eunuch began with a warm-up called "nominal congress," which was nothing more than putting the master's penis in his mouth and moving it around. You can do better than that.

Lick your way up his inner thighs while pulling down gently on his scrotum. Use your finger pads to scratch his testicles. Now take his balls carefully into your mouth, one at a time. Roll them around. Gently pull them down with your mouth.

While you're warming up his balls, run your fingers up and down the shaft of his penis, playing him like the treasured instrument he is.

2. Nibble his shaft.

The Kama Sutra advised using teeth to bite. Ouch! Skip the teeth bites and, instead, try this adaptation. Holding his shaft firmly in your hand, wet your lips and cover your teeth with them. Then you can "bite" up and down his shaft with your lips. Finish by "biting" the head of his penis. The head of the penis is his most sensitive erotic area (like the clitoris). Whatever else you do while performing fellatio, remember to keep coming back to the head.

3. Press your lips against his shaft.
   Presumably this was the "let me kiss that boo-boo my teeth made on your penis" move. Plant pressed lips kisses up and down the shaft in the path of your lip bites. Cover the head with pressed lips and lightly suck. Take as much of his penis as you comfortably can into your mouth, but don't stress too much about this. Only the most sensitive top third is really necessary. Suck. Return to pressed kisses around the corona, the thick ridge separating the head from the shaft. Run your finger repeatedly around the corona.

4. Press his penis inside your mouth.
   And now comes the tease: the Kama Sutra version recommends putting the head of his penis into your mouth, pressing you lips around it, and taking it back out.

   Holding the base of his penis firmly in one hand, run your tongue around the head to moisten it. (Or, if his erection is not firm, you can use both hands wrapped around the shaft in an upward twist stroke.) Circle the head with your tongue in a swirling motion, then work your tongue in long strokes up and down his shaft (what I call the Silken Swirl). Now back to the head. Follow the ridge of the corona with your tongue while working the shaft with your hands, the penis sandwiched between them. Swirl your tongue around it. Tongue the corona. Suck the head. Repeat, repeat, repeat.

   Now do at least ten or twenty seconds of this version of the mouth press: repeatedly pull his penis into your mouth and push it out, using suction, while keeping that tongue in motion around the head.

5. Next, it's the pressing kiss (again).
   The Kama Sutra advises pressing your lips against his penis while holding it in your hand. Press your lips against the head of his penis. Kiss with pressed lips down the shaft. Strum your tongue back and forth across the frenulum, that loose section of skin on the underside of the penis, where the head meets the shaft—another highly sensitive place.

6. Rub the penis.
   Specifically, the Kama Sutra says to touch the penis all over with your tongue. Using broad strokes, run your tongue up and down the shaft. Now tongue his balls. Pay special attention to the raphe, the visible line along

Whether you're performing fellatio or cunnilingus, you need a wet mouth. Keep a glass or carafe of water by the bed. Sip as needed.

Wine or another alcoholic beverage might seem like a sophisticated alternative to water—but save it for after sex. Alcohol dehydrates the body.

the center of the scrotum, an area of the male anatomy that women often overlook. The skin of the scrotum is very sensitive, similar to a woman's labia. Move your tongue back to the shaft and use your thumb to stroke the raphe. Alternate the broad tongue strokes with sucking the head of his penis.

7. Suck the penis.
The Kama Sutra recommends putting half his penis into your mouth and sucking. As mentioned earlier in this section, half isn't necessary, especially if he is large. You have better control over sucking and can keep your tongue moving on the head if you only take the first third of his penis into your mouth. Alternate sucking with the silken swirl (described in step 4), swirling your tongue around the head.

8. Swallow the penis.
The Kama Sutra then describes taking the whole penis into your mouth as if swallowing it. In the modern vernacular, that means perform the Deep Throat. It's a showy move—if you can do it without gagging—but not necessary. Here are some options to try.

• Deep Throat Option 1: Position yourself so that his ejaculate will shoot straight down your throat. Lie on your back with your head off the bed so that your mouth and throat form a smooth line. Have him straddle your face. Swallowing his semen is the inevitable conclusion.

• Deep Throat Option 2: Take as much of his penis into your mouth as you can comfortably handle. Suck it in; push it out. After several of these deeper sucks, concentrate on the head of his penis. As you are sucking him, work one thumb or finger (of the hand firmly holding his penis) up and down the shaft. You can swallow or let the semen dribble discreetly out of your mouth. Apply gentle pressure with your thumb or finger to his perineum when you want him to come—or, if he needs more encouragement, press up firmly against the space between his anus and testicles with the side of your hand, with your thumb pressed against his perineum. (This doesn't work for all men, but it is effective for many.) When he's near ejaculation, take his pelvis in both hands and rock him toward you so that he goes deeper into your mouth.

✌ FUSION TANTRA TECHNIQUE: DON'T NEGLECT HIS G-SPOT
The perineum, that area an inch or so in size between the anus and the base of the scrotum, is an area of men's bodies that is more neglected than the raphe. Rich in nerve endings, the perineum is the second-most-important touch zone for some men—right after the head of the penis. Stroke it lightly, alternate that with gentle pressure from your thumb—and see what happens.

Why is the perineum so important? It links to his G-spot. His G-spot is located inside his body behind the perineum. Pressing the perineum with your thumb or finger will likely stimulate his G-spot. If it doesn't, you can also insert a finger inside his anus and make that same come-hither gesture you used to find your own G-spot. (Be gentle. This is not a prostate exam.)

Many men love G-spot stimulation, but some hate it. You should know how your man feels about a finger in his anus before you put one there.

⚘ ESSENTIAL FUSION TANTRA TECHNIQUE: **THE RESTORATIVE KISS**

You won't find this in the Kama Sutra either, but combining fellatio with a hand job is a no-fail sex technique for restoring a flagging penis, arousing a tired lover, or finishing off your man when you are tired and don't want to play anymore. Here's how it works:

1. Hold his penis firmly in one hand.

2. Take the first third into your mouth and work the remaining two-thirds of the shaft with your hand as you swirl your tongue around the head of the penis to lubricate it.

3. Use the fingers of your other hand to tickle his perineum lightly.

4. Use one hand to make a circular twisting motion up the shaft of his penis as soon as he has a firm erection. (Never twist down.)

5. Swirl your tongue around the corona as you are doing that. (The corona is that ridge separating the shaft from the head of the penis.) Pay particular attention to the frenulum (the small piece of skin where the head meets the shaft).

6. Alternate the swirl with the butterfly flick—flicking your tongue back and forth across the corona.

7. Continue the hand move while taking his testicles into your mouth, one at a time, and sucking lightly.

8. Flick your tongue lightly across his perineum.

9. Go back to the head of his penis and alternate swirling, flicking, and sucking.

10. Don't take his penis too far into your mouth or you won't be able to pull off the suction. Continue until he reaches orgasm.

Cunnilingus

The Kama Sutra instructions for fellatio are minimal at best. But there are no detailed instructions for performing cunnilingus! The original writings on Tantra are equally silent on the subject. Yes, the feminine divine was worshipped. Men were taught to give women pleasure in bed. And, yes, there are references to sacred fluids—specifically male ejaculate, "female ejaculate," and the mingled fluids of a man and a woman making love. All things considered, Tantra was a feminist philosophy for its time. But intercourse was the central sex act at that time.

Most of the practitioners, and probably a high percentage of the teachers, of Neo-Tantra would be surprised to learn that. Cunnilingus is part of their skills set. And it is part of Fusion Tantra, too.

Occasionally a man will tell me that he wants to perform cunnilingus on his woman but she "doesn't like it." Some women do feel uncomfortable letting go in orgasm that way. And some women have issues about how their vagina tastes or smells. But most of the time when a woman says she "doesn't like it," she means she hasn't liked the way her previous partners have performed cunnilingus. Or maybe no one has ever fully aroused her or brought her to orgasm via a skilled tongue. And she doesn't really believe any man can.

The first mistake men make is in going straight for her genitals. You can unzip a man's pants and take his cock into your mouth without any preliminaries, but women generally want to be kissed on their mouth before you put your mouth somewhere else. Start making love to her from the top by expertly kissing her (see page 78). Stroke, massage, nibble, suck, kiss, and lick her body until she is aroused. If she has sensitive breasts or nipples, devote a lot of attention to them. Massage her aureoles with flat, open palms. Gently pull and twist her nipples.

When she is breathing heavily, lick and kiss slowly down from her navel to her vulva. Now lick the line of flesh between her pelvis and thighs. Kiss and lick up and down one inner thigh to the area behind her knees. Now do the same to the other thigh.

Use a small vibrator to stimulate her clitoris while you're kissing and licking her thighs.

Kneel before her. She is ready to be worshipped.

HOW TO ROCK HER WORLD

When performing oral sex on her, she should be in a comfortable position with legs open, knees bent, feet flat, or legs outstretched and open to a V. You can lie or kneel between her legs or come in from the side and wrap one of her legs around your shoulder.

If she is enthusiastic about cunnilingus, she might straddle your face and lower her clitoris to your mouth. A lot of women love this position because it puts them in control of the stimulation they receive.

1. Part her labia gently. Holding the lips open with two fingers of one hand, lift the clitoral hood with the other hand. If her clitoris is well back inside the hood, gently run your fingers along the side of the hood to expose her clitoris. (If she has a deeply set clitoris, you might have to keep one hand in this position until she reaches orgasm.)

2. Use long, broad tongue strokes and lick the skin along the sides, above, and below her clitoris.

3. Don't overlook the U-spot; some women are sensitive to touch just above the urethra, so that can be a potential erogenous zone.

4. Vary your tongue strokes. Press the flat of your tongue against her clitoris and stay still while she moves against you. Circle her clitoris with the tip of your tongue.

5. Insert two fingers into her vagina as you're licking her. Stroke her AFE zone (across from the G-spot, see page 92) until she is wet.

6. Purse your lips around the sides of her clitoris and gently suck. Alternate sucking her clitoris with licking the skin around it.

7. Stroke your fingers inside her vagina, back and forth from the AFE to the G-spot. Pay attention to her responses. Does she pull back when you are licking the clitoris directly (and sucking it)? She probably doesn't like to have her clitoris directly stimulated. It might be too sensitive for the direct approach. On the other hand, is she pulling your head into her body and gyrating her hips wildly? Your technique meets with her approval.

8. Cover her clitoris and surrounding area with your mouth and suck when she is near orgasm.

9. Stimulate her G-spot (if she is G-spot responsive) by pressing repeatedly and lightly against it with your fingertip.

10. Pull your fingers out if she isn't responding to that. Instead, stimulate her labia with your hand. Some women might prefer that you stroke her inner thighs or tease her nipples. Alternate the stimuli, but, of course, leave anything that doesn't get a response out of the rotation.

    Keep your mouth around her clitoris and surrounding area until she has reached orgasm.

Essential Fusion Tantra Tip: The Flick Trick

Even your best move won't work on every woman. Add some variety to your tongue strokes. Keep in mind that the exaggerated licking you see in porn films is a theatrical effect. It looks great on film, but it doesn't do much for the woman actually receiving cunnilingus. In reality, women like much more delicate strokes! Try using only the tip of your tongue to flick back and forth rapidly along the shaft of her clitoris and its tip. Tip flicking sends some women over the top (and is too intense for others). When she is approaching orgasm, tentatively flick back and forth across the top of the clitoris. If she's into it, keep flicking.

MULTIPLE CUNNILINGUS ORGASMS

Once might not be enough. Many women like to have their first orgasm via cunnilingus and then have another orgasm during intercourse. But some women only have multiple orgasms through cunnilingus. Pay attention to her responses. Is she momentarily too sensitive for touch? Or is she finished with the oral part of this event and ready to move on? Give her a minute. Shift your attention from the clitoris to the surrounding area and the vulva. See how she responds. If her hips are still gyrating beneath your mouth and she's got her hands in your hair, she might want more.

❧ FUSION TANTRA TECHNIQUE: **MULTIPLE CUNNILINGUS ORGASM TECHNIQUE #1—THE FLICKERING FLAME**

With apologies to Elton John for the analogy here, this one's a classic. Here's how it works:

1. Pretend the tip of your tongue is a candle flame flickering in the wind. Move your flame/tongue rapidly around the sides of her clitoris and above and below it. Flick across the tiny shaft.

2. Lick the sides of her clitoris in slow, even strokes when she starts to orgasm. As you feel the orgasm subside, return to the fast flicking until she begins to come again.

❧ FUSION TANTRA TECHNIQUE: **MULTIPLE CUNNILINGUS ORGASM TECHNIQUE #2—THE COMBINATION PLAY**

While you are stroking her clitoris and surrounding area with your tongue, add manual stimulation to take her even higher.

1. Use your fingertips to create light circular motions on her vulva.

2. Part her labia. Stroke the outside lips.

3. Curve one or two fingers, and use the space between knuckle and joint to massage her inner and outer lips in a back-and-forth motion. Gauge the pressure to fit her response. Massage her labia and work back to her anus.

4. Alternate the massage with rotating your thumb or first finger around her clitoris, switching between a clockwise and a counterclockwise motion.

5. Now add this: Stroke down with one finger on either side of her clitoris. Rotate. Stroke down.

   And keep your tongue in motion!

❧ FUSION TANTRA TECHNIQUE: MULTIPLE CUNNILINGUS ORGASM TECHNIQUE #3—A STRONGER TOUCH

Some women need or prefer a stronger touch after their first orgasm. Here's a method for doing that, if it suits your partner:

1. Put the tip of your tongue against the shaft of her clitoris.

2. Move your head back and forth, holding your tongue steady while you move your head.
   This next move is not for everyone, but if she likes direct clitoral stimulation, it could be a hit:

3. Take her clitoris between two fingers and gently rotate as you lick the surrounding tissue or even move your tongue down to her labia.

4. Return to holding your tongue against her clitoris and moving your head.

G-SPOT CUNNILINGUS/MANUAL ORGASMS

No, you can't reach her G-spot with your tongue. You can, however, add manual G-spot stimulation to cunnilingus, thus creating an explosive blended orgasm in a woman whose G-spot is responsive.

❧ FUSION TANTRA TECHNIQUE: THE ORAL/G-SPOT DOUBLE PLAY

As you are licking and sucking her clitoris and surrounding area, add this G-spot stroke:

1. Insert a finger or two into her vagina and massage her G-spot.

2. Try tapping it repeatedly with your fingertip.

3. Rub the spot if she doesn't respond to that tapping. Alternate broad strokes with circular rubbing.

4. Flick your tongue rapidly around her clitoris as you're massaging her G-spot. Don't be surprised if she "ejaculates" (see below) during this orgasm.

FEMALE EJACULATION

Some women are "squirters," at least some of the time. Upon orgasm, they excrete fluid—more than the typical amount of vaginal secretions, and sometimes a lot more. Squirting is most likely to happen with G-spot (or a combination of G-spot/AFE zone stimulation.) Many Western sex experts dismiss the "ejaculate" as nothing but a gush of fluid composed of urine and copious vaginal secretions. There is no question that whatever this fluid is, some women do ejaculate, or squirt, upon orgasm, and it is *not* the female equivalent of seminal fluid.

If it is not ejaculate, then what is it? There is no definitive answer to that. Men ejaculate sperm from the testicles via tubes that go through the prostate gland, where the sperm mixes with seminal fluid. Women do not have a prostate gland. *But* in some women, there is a collection of several masses of tissue strung out along the urinary tract, referred to as the skeen gland. This gland produces a fluid that is neither urine nor vaginal secretions, and it might be the source of the fluid squirted.

ADD THE AFE ZONE TO ORAL PLAY

Across from the G-spot is the AFE (anterior fornix erotic) zone, a small, sensitive patch of textured skin—less rough than the G-spot—at the top of the vagina and closer to the cervix. Stroking the AFE zone makes almost any woman lubricate immediately. To find it, explore the front wall of your vagina with one finger. When you feel moisture forming beneath your finger, you've hit it.

A sexologist in Kuala Lumpur rediscovered this area and named it in 1994. The authors of the Kama Sutra wrote about it thousands of years ago.

ESSENTIAL FUSION TANTRA TECHNIQUE: **PLAY ALL THE NOTES**

While sucking or licking her clitoris, massage the G-spot. Then move to the AFE zone. Stroke that area until you feel lubrication. Now go back to the G-spot. Alternate G-spot and AFE zone stroking (while continuing the mouth action) until she comes in a juicy orgasm.

Mutual Oral Sex: The Famous 69

In the Kama Sutra, when describing the mutual oral sex position, the Congress of a Crow, Vatsyayana wrote: "When a man and woman lie down in an inverted order, with the head of one toward the feet of the other and carry on in this congress, it is called the congress of a crow."

He didn't write much more about the mutual oral sex position known in our time as 69. The significant benefit was thought to be in aligning the lovers' chakras. And, of course, it looked good in Indian erotic miniature paintings.

✂ ESSENTIAL FUSION TANTRA TECHNIQUE: **MAKE 69 WORK FOR YOU**

More of a mutual foreplay technique, 69 is probably not an orgasm position. When you have your lover's genitals in your mouth, you must pay attention to what you're doing and how your lover is responding to that. On the other hand, when your genitals are in your lover's mouth, you want to let go and enjoy. Although everyone likes to tout this one as a really hot position, it can be tough balancing these two elements. While mutual oral sex can be a great turn-on, it's not easy to be the mindful performer and the joyful receiver at the same time.

If you do want to take this position to orgasm for one or both of you, then take turns. One should focus on giving the pleasure while the other is receiving, and then vice versa.

Analingus?

Some years ago, the subject of analingus was introduced on the classic HBO sitcom *Sex and the City* by Miranda (Cynthia Nixon's character), who was having trouble understanding why a new lover wanted to lick her anus. Many people will never understand why a lover would either want to lick an anus or have one licked, but it does appeal to others. The anus is rich in nerve endings. If you aren't turned off by the concept, you will probably enjoy the sensations.

The caveats: Bathe or shower first. And don't move your tongue from her clitoris to her anus. That could spread bacteria.

✂ ESSENTIAL FUSION TANTRA TECHNIQUE: **THE LOWER LICK**

Proceed with caution. Ask your lover if you can insert a lubricated finger into his or her anus. When he (or she) is aroused, move your head down.

Lick his (or her) perineum. Now lick around his anus. (If he pulls away, let it go.) Gently pull his butt cheeks apart to emphasize the round, dark hole. Insert the tip of your tongue in and out of his anus in a rhythmic fashion.

Oral lovemaking skills are key to Fusion Tantra. A well-trained tongue and mouth can take your lover higher than you can get him (or her) on intercourse or manual stimulation alone. And intensifying the sexual experience elevates it to Fusion Tantra levels.

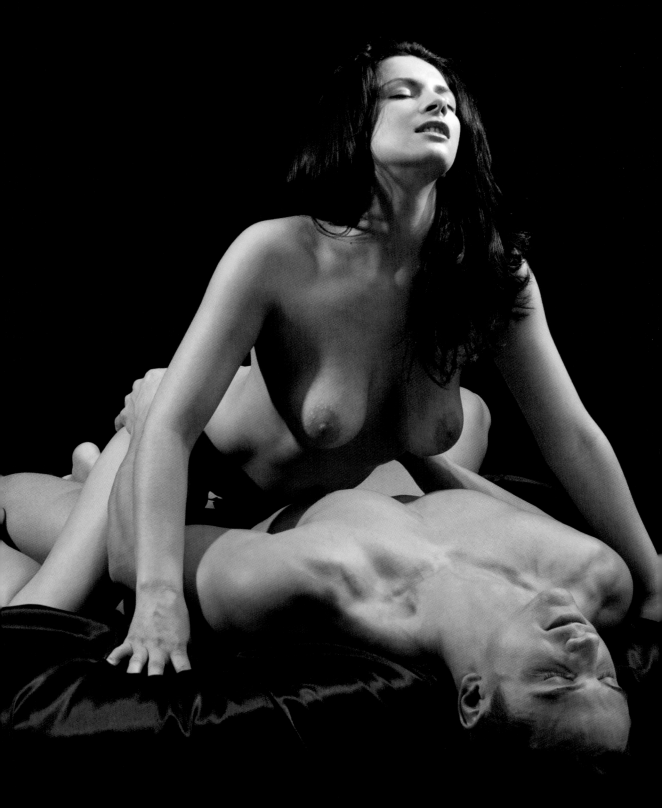

PART 5

The Kama Sutra Positions—New and Improved

Most people think the Kama Sutra is a guide to intercourse positions, but that is only a small (though the most famous) part of the work. Longer sections advise on courtship behavior and describe the "types" of women that men will encounter on their search for a wife. Imagine *Cosmopolitan* magazine as written for men thousands of years ago. No wonder the athletic positions are what survived over time.

I studied a stack of translations, adaptations, and rip-offs of the Kama Sutra before beginning my own work on this book. Some were lush and lavishly photographed; some relied on line drawings and looked almost austere. With each book, I reached a saturation point where what had seemed like innovation became redundancy and then sensory overload: too many intercourse positions, often varying from one to another in only the smallest detail, with emphasis placed on contorted poses; these are not guidelines for real people other than twenty-six-year-old, incredibly fit, nude models.

The books that faithfully reproduce the ancient drawings and statues are beautiful, occasionally rising to the level of an art book. Appreciatethem for the quality of the reproductions and their ability to arouse. And realize that they were created thousands of years ago for that purpose. All the positions were not likely meant to be examples for real couples to use.

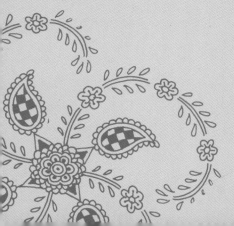

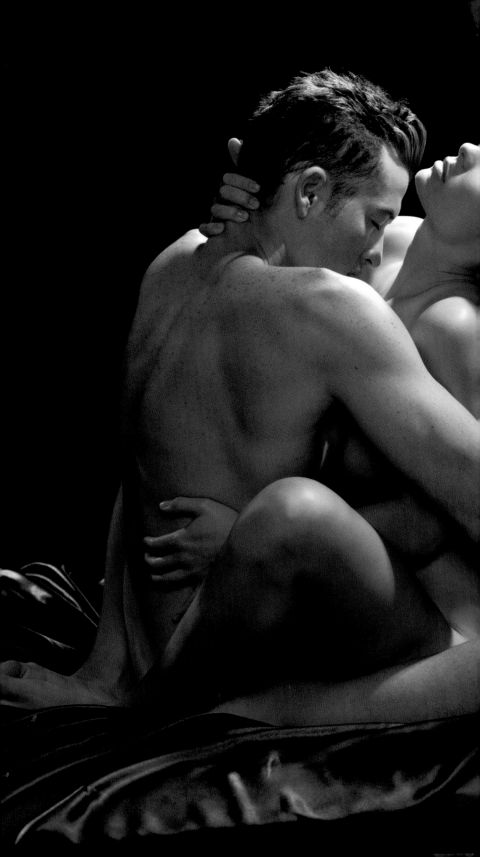

Chapter 13

Discover What the Kama Sutra Got Wrong

The Kama Sutra, the earliest known sex manual, was a collaborative effort—and the collaborators were penis-centric. They also were not as wise about the G-spot and the clitoris as you may have been led to believe. Though the credit is generally given to its famous and gifted editor, Vatsyayana, who lived in India sometime between 100 and 400 a.d., the Kama Sutra was actually written six or seven hundred years before that by many authors. While the book is often regarded as a part of Tantric teaching, it was and still is a physical resource for Tantric sex. And, unlike our sex manuals that are primarily purchased by women and couples, it was aimed at young men of the leisure class (Brahmins), who prided themselves on their sexual knowledge and technique.

The Kama Sutra was also a sexual and social etiquette guide based on the philosophy of "striving to be a superior person." There are three parts to that philosophy: *dharma*, moral responsibility or righteousness; *artha*, the acquisition of riches; and *kama*, the pursuit of a high level of eroticism. All were emphasized in the text. But it's the intercourse positions that have fascinated readers throughout history.

Two other books written a thousand years or more after the Kama Sutra are also regarded as classics: the *Ananga Ranga*, which also originated in India, and *The Perfumed Garden*, an Arabian sex manual that, in addition to giving sex advice, included sections on sensual foods and aphrodisiacs. It also created "types" of men and women that would be familiar to women's magazine readers today. The *Ananga Ranga* was written for later generations of Indians and reflected the more sexually conservative cultural attitudes of the times. While the Kama Sutra spoke to single Indian men, the *Ananga Ranga* addressed married men, such as by giving advice on how to keep the boredom out of their sex lives without taking lovers.

Beyond the Kama Sutra

Now, from the ancient history of the Kama Sutra, let's get back to the present. Fusion Tantra picks up where the Kama Sutra leaves off—and incorporates what the Kama Sutra leaves out. The Kama Sutra was relentlessly penis-centric and all about intercourse. Sure, the Kama Sutra's writers were ahead of their time in a sense because they found the G-spot. They even recognized the G-spot's importance, but (in those pre-vibe centuries) they couldn't imagine how anything but a big penis could hit it properly. It's no surprise, then, that one of the Kama Sutra's primary concerns was how to make small penises feel bigger. They underestimated the clitoris, too. In Fusion Tantra, there is more to the G-spot than this—read on and see.

✎ ESSENTIAL FUSION TANTRA TECHNIQUE: **EMPLOYING THE G-SPOT**

Yes, that place referred to as the sacred spot in Tantra texts correlates to the modern G-spot. The G-spot was rediscovered by Beverly Whipple in the 1980s. It is named after the German physician Ernst Grafenberg, who "discovered" it in the 1940s, but this place was familiar territory to the Indian authors of the Kama Sutra five thousand years earlier. And each one of us feels like an explorer when we find our own.

I don't know whether controversy surrounded the sacred spot, but it certainly has followed the G-spot. Through the years, some experts have debunked its importance, even denied its existence, while others have endowed it with almost sexual superpower. Does it exist? Is it important? Can you tell the difference between a G-spot orgasm and a clitoral orgasm? There are no correct answers to any of these questions, including "Does it exist?" Some women have tried and failed to find their G-spot. We can conclude that it doesn't exist for them. Search for yours. If you find it, you decide how important it is and whether or not your G-spot orgasm is different from other orgasms.

First, if you haven't done so already, find the G-spot. Some women find it by lying on their backs; others reach it on their stomachs; and some have to squat. Once you've located yours, try the following:

1. Place your palm down on your vulva.

2. Insert a lubricated finger or two into your vagina and make the come hither gesture. Explore. Do you feel a rough patch on the upper wall of

your vagina? That's your G-spot, and it gets engorged with blood when you are aroused.

Now play with the spot once you find it.

3. Use your fingers, a G-spot vibe, or a regular vibe with a G-spot attachment. (I prefer the vibe because it's more comfortable than stretching my fingers up there.) The tip of the vibe should point up toward the spot.

4. Experiment with pressure and strokes. Many women like firm G-spot pressure and short, repetitive strokes right on the spot. Others like to circle around it. You might come from G-spot stimulation, or you might need to add clitoral stimulation. You might even ejaculate. (Although this doesn't happen to all women, some women experience a squirting of liquid that might be part vaginal secretions, part urine. See page 91 for more on this.)

Rock 'n' Roll That Pelvis (and His Size Won't Matter)

Maybe the most desirable penis is longer and thicker than average. Nevertheless, a woman can still get what she wants and needs during intercourse with Mr. Average Man, especially if she is flexible.

Women need to be more flexible than men to get the most out of intercourse. His movement is thrusting in and out with the easily reachable goal of getting friction to the head of his penis. She has more paths to orgasm (see page 38) than he does. And she can dramatically affect the coital sensations by shifting her body a few inches in a different direction. Sometimes the difference between orgasm and "almost" is a small matter of gyrating her hips in a different track.

Women, before you get into any position, loosen your pelvis. These exercises are adapted from yoga exercises I learned in class, from a friend, or in a textbook. They not only help make your pelvis more flexible but they also help you feel sexier.

✵ FUSION TANTRA EXERCISE: **THE CLASSIC CAT**

Just getting into this position releases some of your pent-up sexual energy.

1. Get down on all fours.

2. Inhale, and get into a swaybacked position by bringing your shoulders up and in and lifting your head.

3. Exhale now, arching your upper back and tucking your pelvis in and under.

4. Draw your diaphragm up and in, and pull your anal muscles up and in.

5. Bring your chin down to your chest.

6. Meow or roar; paw the ground with your hands. Repeat this several times.

✷ FUSION TANTRA EXERCISE: **THE SEXY SQUAT**

This one is a simple move, but it can be a challenge to hold. Don't worry; it's worth it.

It's good for your thighs and butt, as well as your sex life.

1. Stand with your feet shoulder-width apart and slowly lower your butt as if you were going to sit in a chair.

2. Squeeze your PC muscle and the muscles in your buttocks as you rise back up.

3. Do three times daily.

✷ FUSION TANTRA EXERCISE: **THE SEAT**

1. Sit back on your heels and reach your arms forward.

2. Hold for one minute.

3. Sit up and lean back as far as you can, with your hands on the floor behind you for support.

4. Hold for one minute.

5. Do three times daily.

✷ FUSION TANTRA EXERCISE: **THE PELVIC HOT THRUST**

You'll turn yourself on doing this one.

1. Stand in front of a full-length mirror, with your arms hanging loosely at your sides.

2. Breathe deeply through your mouth, all the way down to your belly.

3. Imagine that you are breathing air into your pelvis and your vagina.

4. Breathe it back out again.

5. Rock back and forth with the movement generated in your pelvis. The rocking should remain centered in your pelvis.

6. Keep your chest and back relaxed, not rigid.

7. Rock forward as you inhale.

8. Let your pelvis rock backward on the exhalation.

9. Rock back and forth for three to four minutes.

How Important Is Penis Size?

According to the Kama Sutra, it was of utmost importance. A man with a small penis was considered lacking, and positions were developed to maximize his potential. But in our day, the politically correct answer is: penis size is not important.

Aesthetically, penis size is very important to some women—just as aesthetically, breast size is very important to some men. But it doesn't make that much difference in lovemaking. First, the overwhelming majority of men are average size. (According to The Kinsey Institute, roughly 2 percent of men are nine inches and over, with another 2 percent being three inches or under. Everyone else falls into the middle range.) Second, small penises expand more with erection than large ones do—somewhat leveling the playing field, so to speak. And, third, good lovers can make their body parts work together, regardless of size.

If a woman has a strong PC muscle, she can wrap her vagina around a penis—large, medium, or small—and make the flexing and releasing of her muscle feel good for both of them. Intercourse positions can be adapted to create satisfactory thrusting sensations with a penis of any size. The bottom line is: two-thirds of women do not reach orgasm via intercourse alone. They need direct clitoral stimulation. No matter how big the penis, it won't get her there without some help.

Some women instinctively maximize direct contact of his pubic bone and her vulva in an intercourse style that can best be described as "grinding"—and that works well with a small penis. That allows them to reach orgasm without using hands (not that there is anything wrong with using hands). Positions that open her legs and vulva wide are good grinding positions. Side positions and the Starfish (see page 130) create favorable stimulation angles for a short but thick penis. No matter what his penis size is, she (and he) can work with it.

We can give the authors of the Kama Sutra credit for making a woman's pleasure the highest priority. But they were men—and men who were obsessed with their penis size and their performance. Thus, they assumed a woman's pleasure was determined by how well they used their object of obsession. They didn't grasp the full significance of her clitoris or even her G-spot. Fusion Tantra gives all due respect (even worship) to the male organ, but it doesn't hold it responsible for women's orgasms.

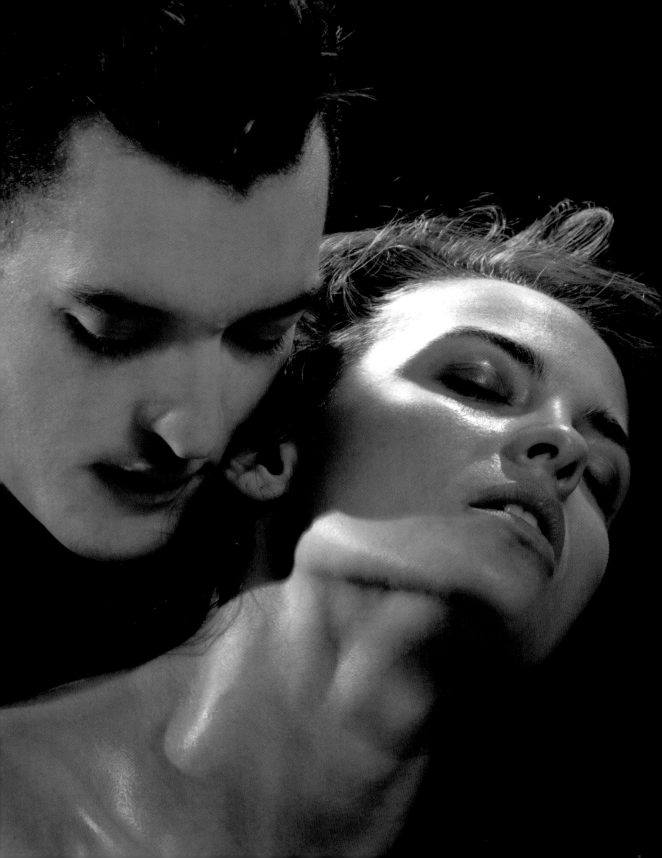

Chapter 14

The Twelve Fusion Tantra Positions Your Sex Life Needs

There are six basic groups of intercourse positions: woman on top, man on top, rear entry, side by side, sitting, and standing. Every position, including the most contorted gymnastic poses of the Kama Sutra, is a variation on one of these themes. Dr. Alfred Kinsey used the six basics as categories in the sexual behavior questionnaires that formed the basis of his landmark books on male and female sexuality.

If you asked the average person how many positions were described in the original Kama Sutra, he or she would most likely guess too high. The correct answer is thirty-five—and even that number contains several repetitive poses where the difference from one pose to the next is slight enough to require a second or third glance to find it. All thirty-five positions fit into one of the six categories.

Rather than striving for mastery of many positions, learn how to do the basics in two ways each—and then add creative adaptations as your moods, bodies, or partners change.

Woman on Top (Female Superior)

This was the most common position in ancient Greek and Roman civilizations, as well as in India and China. Woman on Top is also the basic intercourse position often touted in our day as "best for female orgasm." Kinsey found it a favorite among educated and upper-middle-class people.

With the greatest possible ability to control the depth of penetration and the speed of thrusting, a woman has maximum orgasm advantage when she's on top. She or he can stimulate her clitoris and/or breasts more easily than in other positions. And that explains why Woman on Top is as popular (if not more) among younger lovers than Man on Top, once the ubiquitous intercourse position among Western couples.

FUSION TANTRA POSITION #1: SHE'S ON TOP

Adapted from "Pair of Tongs," a Kama Sutra position, She's on Top is based on the classic configuration: he lies on his back; she sits astride. A strong PC muscle is mandatory, not merely helpful, here.

Here are some of the benefits of She's on Top:

- It works for urgent as well as playful sex.

- It is good when he's tired or wants to relinquish control.

- It is visually stimulating for him—a plus if he's not feeling as energetic as she is.

- It provides maximum indirect clitoral stimulation by his penis.

- It allows him to play with her breasts and genitals.

- It gives her freedom of movement, especially if her partner is much larger.

- It is suited to any penis size, because she controls the angle and depth of penetration.

- It increases G-spot stimulation.

The Setup

Here's how it works:

1. He lies on his back, with one or both knees bent.
2. She either squats on her haunches and lowers herself onto his penis, or sits astride him, knees bent, with her hands on his chest.
3. She pulls him inside her as she lowers herself on to him, squeezing her PC muscle around his penis. Doing this also stimulates her G-spot.

The Fusion Tantra Difference

The critical difference between She's on Top and the traditional female superior position is that she limits her up-and-down movements and controls the action primarily by flexing her PC muscle and thighs.

This position was given its Kama Sutra name, "Pair of Tongs," because she squeezes his penis, lifting it inside her and pushing it out—as if her vagina were a pair of tongs plucking him.

Variations

1. She leans further forward, even letting her breasts touch his chest if she wants. On the downward stroke, she grinds her clitoris into his pubic bone, thus adding direct clitoral stimulation.
2. She leans backward, shifting her weight to her hands placed behind her. While dramatically changing the angle of penetration with this move, she also creates an exciting visual for her man, as well as the opportunity for him to stimulate her clitoris with his fingers.
3. This variation takes Variation #2 a little further and requires flexibility on the woman's part. He straightens his legs on the bed and props himself up on one or both elbows. She leans backward so that she is lying on top of his legs, her back slightly arched. Again, he can enjoy the view from this angle and also stimulate her manually.

Top, Position #1;
Bottom left, Variation #2; Bottom right, Variation #3

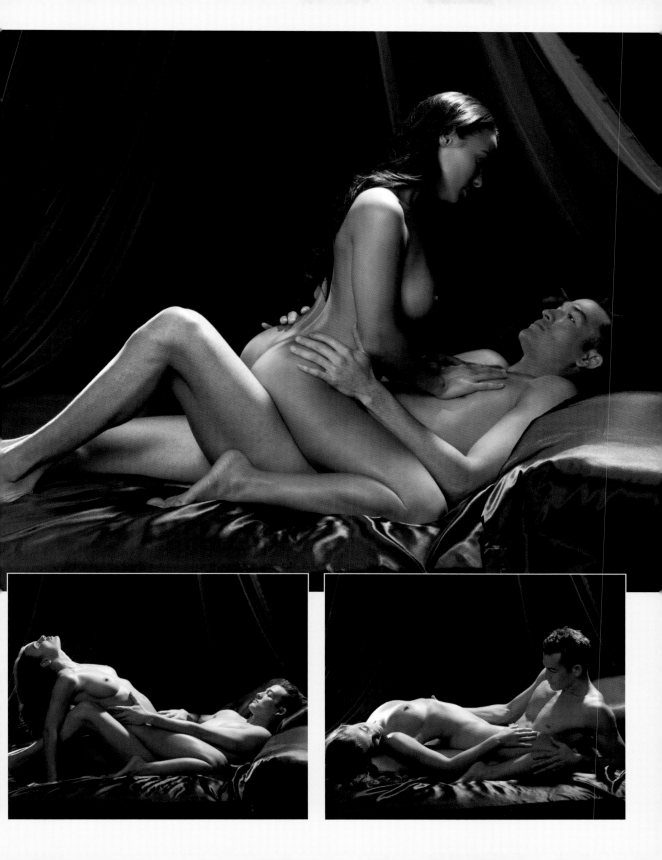

FUSION TANTRA POSITION #2:
REVERSE COWGIRL

Known as "Mare's Position" in the Kama Sutra, the Reverse Cowgirl is the flip side of She's on Top: he lies on his back; she sits astride him facing the opposite way.

Here are some of the benefits of the Reverse Cowgirl:

- It can be more comfortable if his penis is large.

- It is a good position for angry sex—there is no eye contact!

- It also works well when you're more into the mechanics of sex, rather than the emotion.

- It lets her thrust vigorously by holding onto his calves or ankles and pushing back and forth against him.

- It shows off a shapely ass.

The Setup

Here's how it works:

1. He lies down flat or with his back supported by a stack of pillows against the headboard (in the same slouched-down position he might use to read in bed).

2. She sits astride him with her knees bent as she faces his feet.

The Fusion Tantra Difference

Again, she uses her PC muscle to pull him in and push him out—but she augments that flex/release with more active thrusting movements than she does in the previous position.

Variations

1. He adjusts the angle of his back (propped against pillows) until he can comfortably reach around to her genitals as she rides him. Arching her back slightly, she moves up and down while he reaches around her to massage her clitoris.

2. She elongates her body so that her legs are almost stretched out alongside his body. Lying with her head between his legs, she controls thrusting primarily through PC flex/release.

*Top, Position #2;
Bottom, Variation #2*

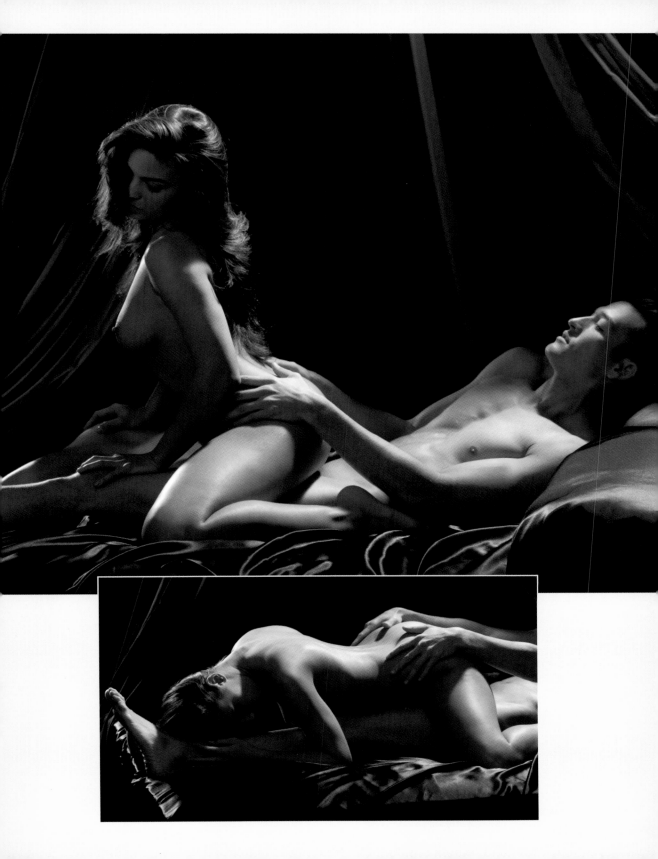

Man on Top (Missionary)

The position most often associated with intercourse, Western style, is Man on Top, or missionary position. According to legend, the natives of the Pacific Islands named the position after the missionaries who had intercourse this way only because they considered other positions "sinful."

Despite its past reputation, Man on Top is still a much-loved position. Sex surveys (such as recent ones on iVillage and in *Marie Claire* magazine) consistently rank missionary as one of women's top two favorite positions. It's a good position for closeness and emotional connection, and it's also a good position physically because it allows for hard thrusting.

FUSION TANTRA POSITION #3: THE EASY LAY

Inspired by one of the Kama Sutra twists on the missionary position, the Easy Lay is based on this simple configuration: she lies on her back; he faces her.

Here's what's great about the Easy Lay:

- It's comfortable for both partners.

- It allows her to vary the coital dynamics by opening her legs wide or closing them around his waist.

- It enables both to utilize PC flex/release to greatest advantage for controlling thrusting.

- It gives her more effective G-spot stimulation than the missionary position does.

The Setup

Here's the walk-through:

1. She lies on her back; he straddles her on his knees. Her hands clasp his thighs.
2. She arches her back and brings her legs over his thighs (reversing the straddle). Her feet are flat on the bed with her body forming a line from shoulders to bent knees.

3. He supports her by holding onto her hips. Or, if she can support herself by putting her weight on his thighs and her feet, he can use his free hands to massage her clitoris and/or breasts.
4. She affects the thrusting dynamics by squeezing her thighs together or by wrapping one leg around his waist as he thrusts.

The Fusion Tantra Difference

Thighs take this position beyond the ordinary. By using her thighs to affect coital dynamics or his thighs to balance her weight, she is opening up the position.

Variations

1. She pulls her knees up toward her chin. The higher her knees are, the deeper the penetration will be. If she puts her feet on his shoulders, he will penetrate her more deeply and she will get G-spot stimulation.
2. This variation, adapted from the Kama Sutra position "Tail of the Ostrich," looks like it will require gymnastic ability, but it really doesn't. Facing her, he is on his knees with his back straight (in other words, standing on his knees). She is lying down facing him. He lifts her legs up to his shoulders. She slides up his body as he does this. Her weight is supported on her shoulders in what looks like a yoga shoulder-stand position. With his erection pointing down toward her vagina, he enters her. He wraps his arms around her thighs for support as he thrusts. The position is difficult to sustain for prolonged intercourse. Use it to ignite arousal. Then fold into the Easy Lay.

Center, Position #3;
Inset, Variation #2

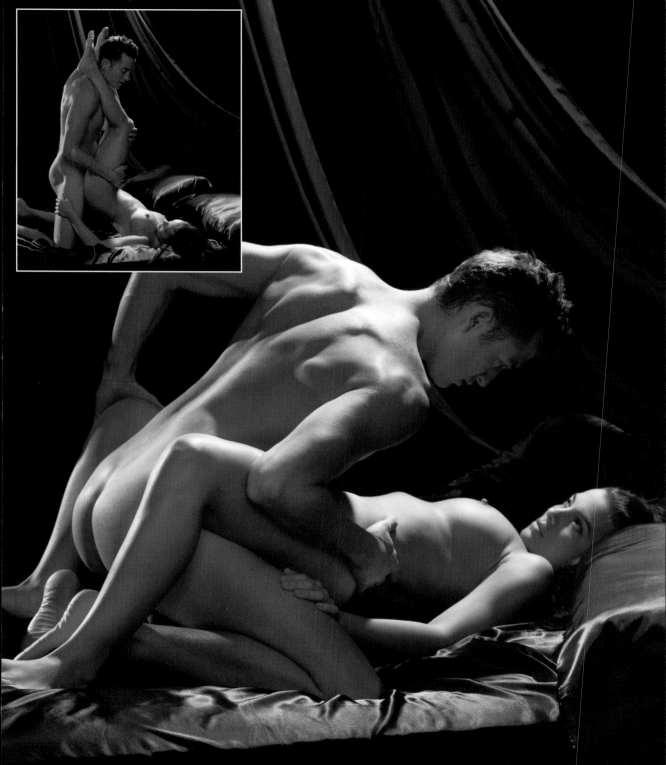

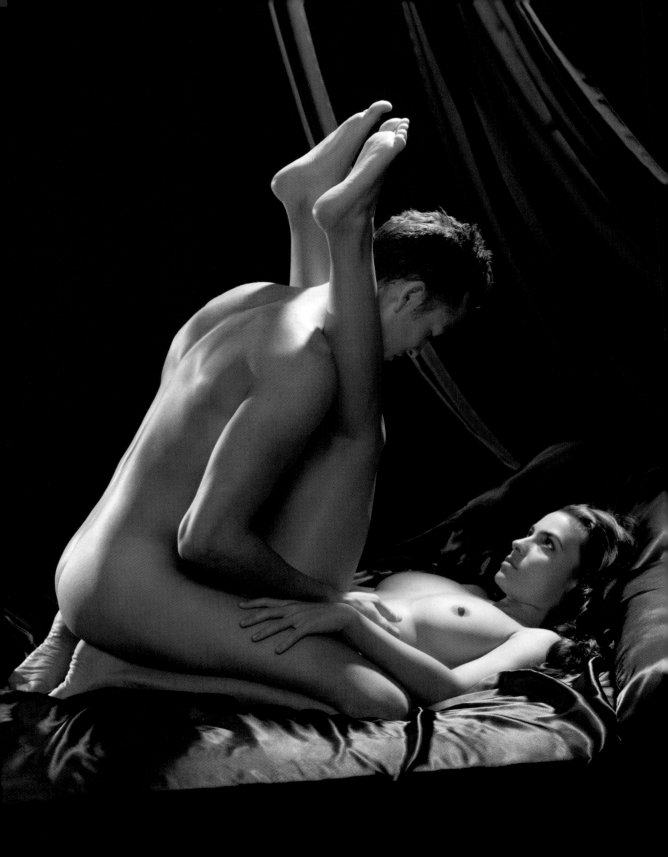

FUSION TANTRA POSITION #4: LEGS UP

Adapted from the Kama Sutra's "Rising Position," Legs Up is again based on this simple model: she lies on her back, legs up; he faces her.

Here are the pros to Legs Up:

- It makes her vagina feel tighter to him.

- It allows her to use her thighs in thrusting, which is helpful if her PC muscle isn't well toned.

- It works even if their body sizes are disproportionate.

The Setup

Here is a walk-through of the position:

1. She lies on her back, raises her legs straight up, and puts them over his shoulders as he kneels in front of her.
2. He might have to keep his knees close together or spread wide so that her body is between his knees. (This depends on their body sizes and states of flexibility.)
3. Her legs may be open and outstretched or pulled together at the knees (which should be roughly at his chest level).
4. He thrusts while leaning slightly forward, balancing his weight on his knees with his hands placed on either side of her body. Or he thrusts in an upright position, clasping her legs for leverage and support.
5. Her movement is limited, but she can influence thrusting by flexing her PC muscle and squeezing her thighs together.

The Fusion Tantra Difference

Here, the woman can influence thrusting by flexing her PC muscle and squeezing her thighs together. This gives her power in the position and makes orgasm more likely.

Variations

1. The Leg Switch: Called "The Splitting of a Bamboo" in the Kama Sutra, the Leg Switch is like bicycling. Instead of putting both legs over his shoulders, she puts one over and wraps the other around his waist or leaves that leg straight beside him. Periodically, she switches legs, taking the one off his shoulder and moving it around his waist (or beside him) and putting the other leg over his shoulder. As she changes legs, her vagina naturally squeezes his penis.
2. She opens her legs wide. He kneels between them. She wraps her legs around his waist or puts her feet on the bed, knees bent. The wide angle of her hips may make her G-spot and AFE zone (see page 92) more accessible, especially if he has a large penis.

Rear Entry

An unfortunate colloquial name—"Doggy Style"—made this position appear to be politically incorrect back in the (really not-so-far-back) day when anything smacking of male domination seemed like a bad idea. A favorite of many women and men, rear entry is a Kama Sutra basic that was quite popular with the ancient Greeks, too. I sometimes wonder whether it wasn't the original intercourse position. Primates do it this way, and man is a primate. Logically, wouldn't evolution favor an intercourse position that allowed both the man and the woman to keep an eye on the cave door or the jungle perimeter?

Rear-entry positions were prevalent in *The Perfumed Garden*, written in the late fifteenth century by Sheikh Nefzawi (and translated by Sir Richard Burton in the nineteenth century) as a sex advice book for men. He labeled all his intercourse positions as "postures" and simply numbered each. Because he believed that women were best satisfied by a large penis, he paid special attention to developing positions that would afford even the less endowed man the illusion of size.

FUSION TANTRA POSITION #5: THE PRIMAL POSITION

Adapted from the Sixth Posture in *The Perfumed Garden*, the Primal Position is based on this classic configuration: she kneels on all fours; he enters her vagina from behind.

Here are the pluses of the Primal Position:

- It is effective for men with small penises.

- It tightens and elongates the woman's vagina.

- It allows for direct clitoral stimulation.

- It provides G-spot stimulation.

- It affords him a good view of her ass—and an opportunity to administer a few slaps, if desired.

- It is good for urgent sex, or for angry sex, because there is no eye contact.

The Setup
Here are the steps to this position:
1. She kneels on the bed, putting her weight on her arms.
2. He kneels behind her, between her legs. Holding on to her hips, he enters her.
3. He guides her body back and forth on his penis, by holding on to her hips or her waist.
4. She flexes her PC muscle as he pulls her onto his penis, releasing as he pushes her back.

The Fusion Tantra Difference
The distinction between this version and the classic rear entry position is that he's pulling her back and forth onto his penis rather than thrusting into her, creating a different sensation.

Variations
1. Relying less on PC flex/release, he thrusts more vigorously and either he or she strokes her clitoris at the same time.
2. She lowers her chest flat or close to flat to the bed, changing the angle and depth of penetration.

Center, Position #5:
Inset, Variation #2

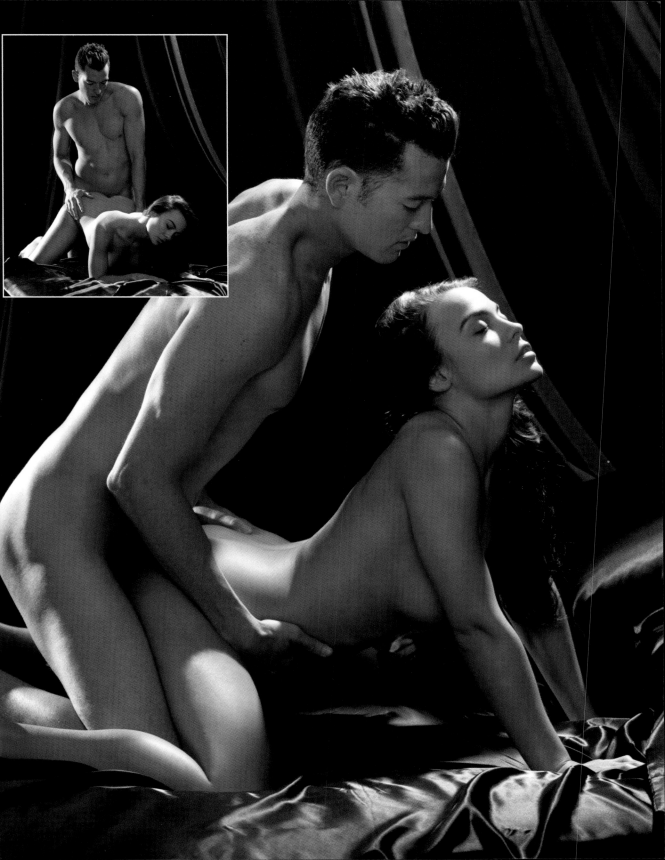

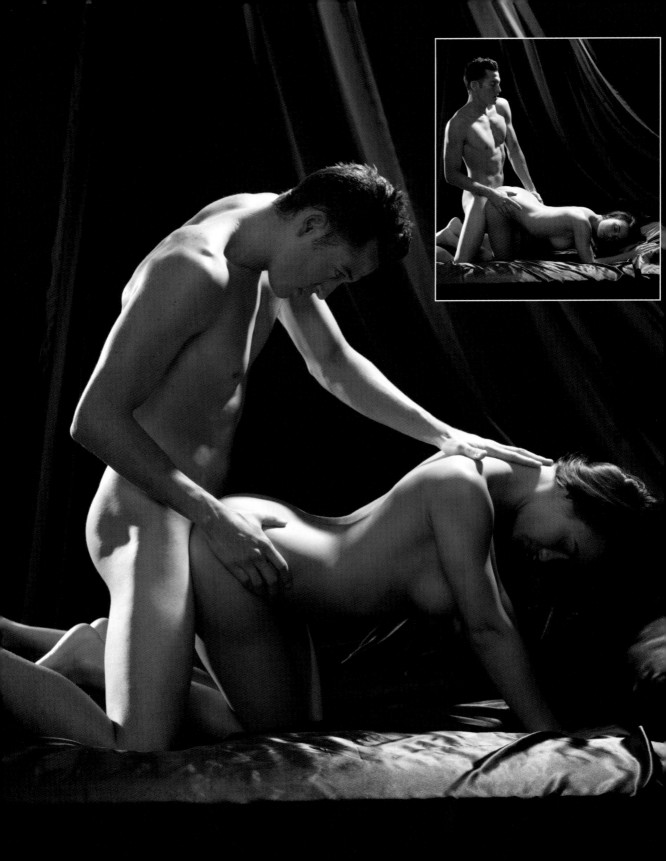

FUSION TANTRA POSITION #6:
THE LAZY PRIMAL

Adapted from the Ninth Posture in *The Perfumed Garden*, the Lazy Primal has this basic configuration: she kneels; he enters her vagina from behind.

The Lazy Primal has these benefits:

- It is effective for men with small penises.

- It tightens and elongates her vagina.

- It provides G-spot stimulation.

- It makes a good quickie position.

The Setup
Here's how this position plays out:

1. She kneels on the floor and lies/drapes the top half of her body across a bed, couch, table, or other surface. Alternatively, if it's more comfortable, she can simply position herself on all fours on the bed.
2. He enters her from behind, while kneeling and straddling her legs.
3. He holds on to her hips as he thrusts vigorously.
4. She pushes back against him. On her forward movement, she can get direct clitoral stimulation from grinding into the mattress or other surface. This is a great position for sex outside the bedroom because it works without removing much clothing except, perhaps, her panties.

The Fusion Tantra Difference
In this position, she gets the additional stimulation she needs to reach orgasm from grinding into the mattress.

Variations

1. She leans forward on her forearms, raising her bottom up against him. This slight variation provides a different angle of penetration. He holds her hips to help regulate his thrusting.
2. He lifts her bottom up so that she is no longer resting on her knees. She supports her weight on her arms. He won't penetrate as deeply in the higher position, making intercourse last longer and/or taking some of the pressure off her if he has a large penis.
3. Assuming a wide-legged crouch rather than kneeling, she leans forward with her forearms resting on a piece of furniture. Her right leg, angled to the side and slightly bent at the knee, is braced against the furniture. Her left leg, also slightly bent, is almost straight behind her. He gets down on his left knee between her legs and puts his right knee under her right thigh to support her. Since he has more freedom of movement than she has, he holds her by the waist, pulling her back and forth in time with his thrusting. (It sounds more complicated than it is.) The position changes the angle of penetration, giving her different sensations.

Center, Position #6;
Inset, Variation #1

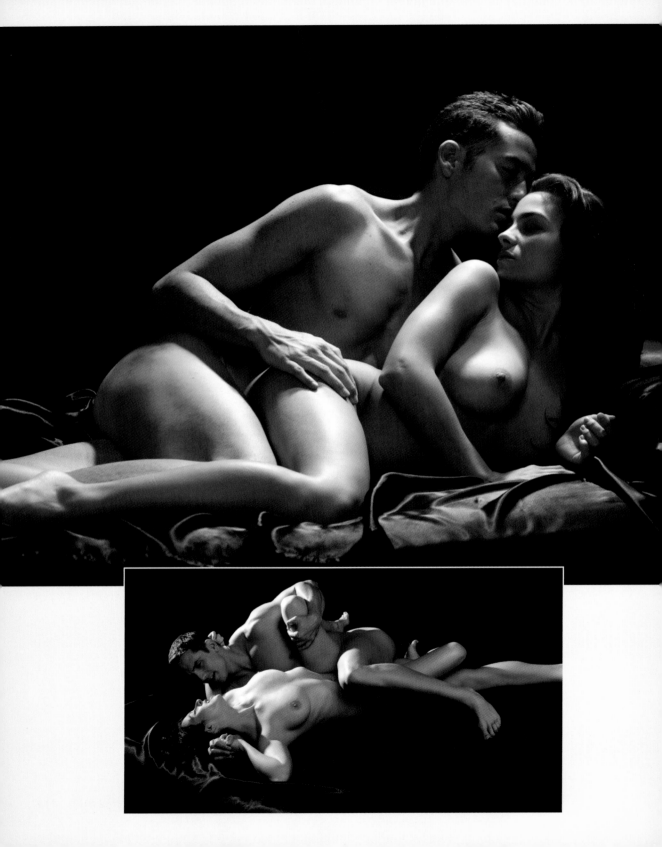

Side by Side

The Roman poet and philosopher Ovid wrote lyrically about the side-by-side position, while twentieth-century French lovers considered it most suited for "the lazy," which we all can be sometimes. Side-by-side positions are great, however, because they are not static—you can start out facing each other, then shift to lying half on your side, half on your back (or your partner can), or move to a spooning position.

Many couples use the side by side as a starter position, for example, when one is awake and ready for sex and the other isn't quite there. It's also a gentle make-up sex position for the couple who doesn't yet want to look one another in the eye.

FUSION TANTRA POSITION #7: SWEET SEX

Adapted from the "Transverse Lute" position in the Kama Sutra, Sweet Sex uses this opening configuration: lying on their sides, he faces her back, in a spooning position. They can shift so that one partner is half on her side, half her on back.

Here are the benefits to Sweet Sex:

- It is good for low-energy sex.

- It is very effective for a short, thick penis.

- It allows easy, direct clitoral stimulation.

- It helps him sustain intercourse longer.

The Setup

A good wake-up sex position, this also works if she wants to pull one more orgasm from an extended lovemaking session. Here's how it works:

1. They wrap their arms around one another in a tight embrace once they are on their sides, facing the same direction.
2. He enters her from behind and flexes his pelvic floor muscles in time with her own PC flexing. All movement is confined to muscle flexing in this one. No thrusting!
3. They may both prop themselves on one elbow and relax their embrace as they flex together. He may hold her by the hip for deeper penetration.

The Fusion Tantra Difference

In this version, she reaches orgasm through flexing her PC muscle.

Variations

1. She raises one leg slightly. To give her extra clitoral stimulation, he also raises one leg and rests it on her thigh and pulls himself higher so that his penis rubs against her clitoris as he flexes.
2. He supports himself on one elbow rather than remaining flat on the bed. He enters her from behind. As he does, she half turns (from the waist) so that they can look into one another's eyes. Their legs stay intertwined and he holds on to her bent leg with his free arm.

Top, Position #7;
Bottom, Variation #2

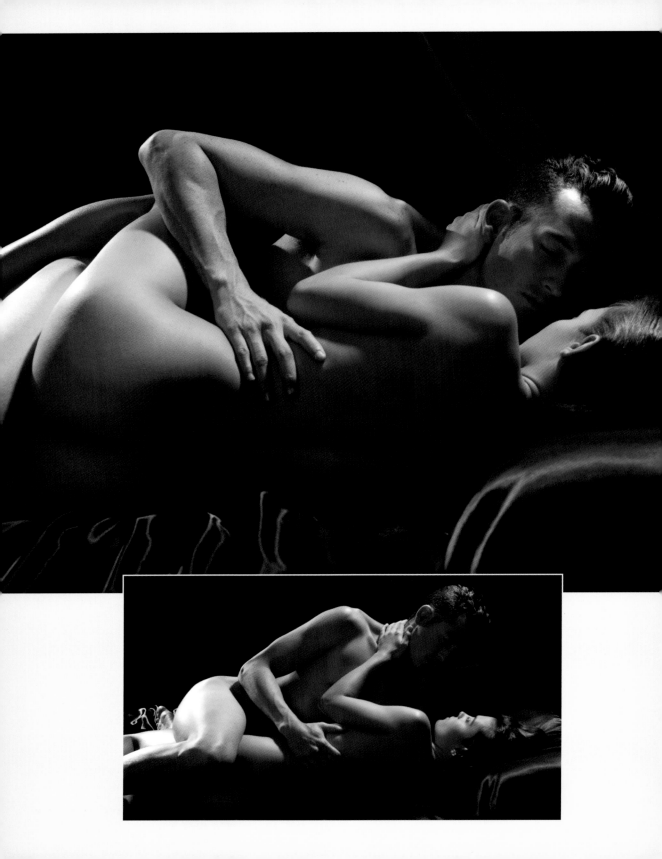

FUSION TANTRA POSITION #8: THE FACE UP

Adapted from the Kama Sutra's "Crab Embrace" position, the Face Up has a simple configuration: lying in one another's arms, the couple faces each other.

The Face Up is great for these reasons:

- It is a romantic way to begin lovemaking.

- It helps lovers who have been apart feel close and connected.

- It affords kissing, face stroking, and cuddling.

- It gives her good clitoral stimulation.

The Setup

Here are the logistics of this one:

1. They lie on their sides, face to face.
2. She has one leg between his and another wrapped around his waist.
3. He inserts his penis inside her.
4. They grind against one another, rather than thrusting, as they kiss, gaze into each other's eyes, and touch and caress one another's bodies.

The Fusion Tantra Difference

With this position, the couple grinds rather than thrusts. And they employ emotional and sensual foreplay techniques during intercourse.

Variations

1. This variation allows for the deepest penetration possible in the side-by-side position; He lies between her thighs. She has one leg beneath his and the other wrapped around his waist.
2. She places one of her legs between his thighs and throws the other leg over his body after he enters her. He rolls over so that he is half on his side and half on his back. She has more freedom of movement and can thrust against their grinding motion.
3. He places one of his thighs around her waist and props himself up on one elbow, gazing down at her. He thrusts in an upward motion.

Top, Position #8;
Bottom, Variation #3

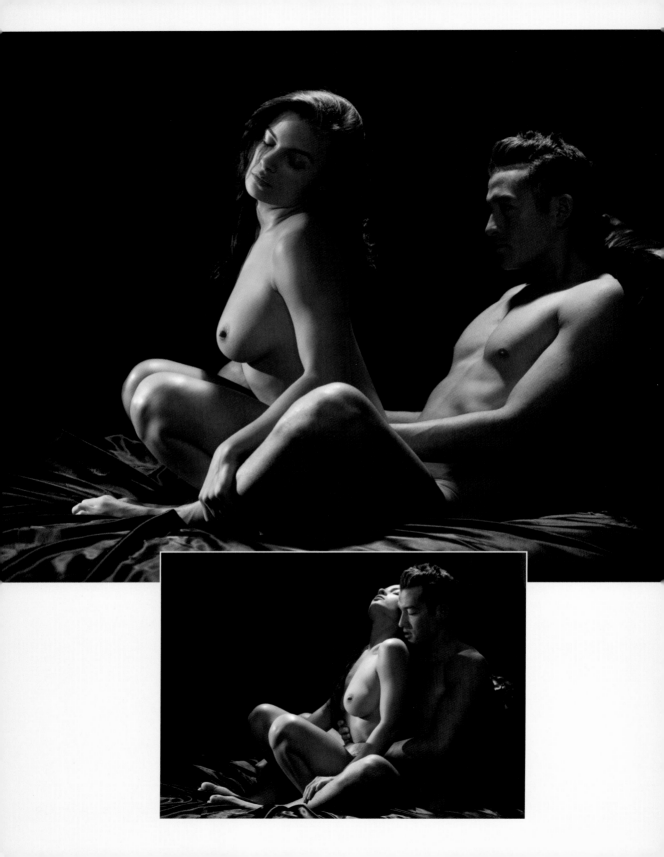

Sitting

If you are familiar with Indian art, you have seen paintings and statues of lovers in the sitting position, with her on his lap. The Hindu elephant god Ganesh frequently made love to his consort in this manner. Thousands of years later, many members of the baby boom and subsequent generations had sex for the first time in a sitting position—in the backseat of a car.

Whether it brings back memories or not, the sitting position is a playful way to have intercourse.

FUSION TANTRA POSITION #9: THE REVERSE SIT

A scaled-down version of a complicated Kama Sutra position called "The Swing," the Reverse Sit is configured like this: He sits up with his legs outstretched. She sits with her back toward him.

Following are the benefits of the Reverse Sit:

- It allows a short penis to penetrate more deeply than most other positions do.

- It limits his thrusting ability to prolong love-making or give one partner time to catch up to the other's arousal level.

- It is a playful way for her to be in charge of the coital dynamics.

The Setup

Here's how it works:

1. He leans back slightly while in a sitting position. His weight is on his hands, which are flat on the bed and positioned comfortably behind him. (Or he can support his back with the headboard or pillows if that feels better.)
2. He bends his legs slightly or stretches them loosely and comfortably out in front of him.
3. With her back to him, she sits down on his erection. Her knees are bent and her legs are between his.
4. She leans forward and braces herself by holding on to his calves or ankles (depending on what feels good).
5. She thrusts back against him as he moves forward into her.

The Fusion Tantra Difference

In the ancient version of this position, he placed his hands well behind his arched back once seated—not so comfortable. Meanwhile, she swiveled her body on his penis, facing from front to back and round again—not so easy. In this adaptation, they are not restricted to rigid poses. Fusion Tantra is more fluid and forgiving of imperfect bodies.

Variations

1. They both sit up straighter so that her back is against his chest. He strokes her clitoris with one hand as she rides up and down on his penis.
2. He sits on a comfortable chair or sofa. She sits on his lap but leans forward, bracing herself on a piece of furniture or with her hands on the floor. He holds her around the waist as she moves her body on his penis.

Top, Position #9;
Bottom, Variation #1

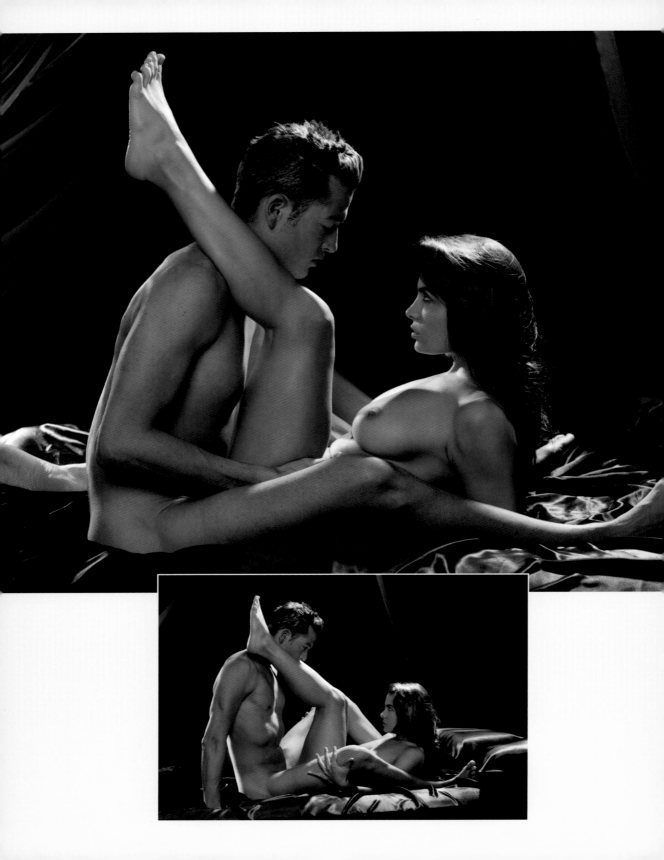

FUSION TANTRA POSITION #10:
THE MOVING SIT

Adapted from the Kama Sutra position called the "Rocking Horse," the Moving Sit has this basic configuration: the couple sit facing one another.

Here are some pros to the Moving Sit:

- It is the most athletic of the twelve Fusion Tantra down-and-dirty positions.

- It allows sexual energy to build slowly.

- It gives him an intimate view of her vagina.

- It requires cooperation—and that makes the lovers more attentive to each other.

The Setup

Here are the steps for the Moving Sit:

1. He sits with his legs stretched wide apart.
2. She faces him and sits between his legs.
3. He clasps her wrists or forearms to support her as she puts one leg over his shoulder.
4. She leans back as he penetrates her, resting her weight on her outstretched arms.
5. They move together gently until both are highly aroused.
6. She lowers her leg from his shoulder and wraps both ankles around his body at chest level.
7. They rock back and forth, while clasping one another's wrists and forearms.

The Fusion Tantra Difference

The chest-level ankle wrap changes the angle of penetration here, increasing arousal and encouraging orgasm to happen faster.

Variations

1. He sits back with his shoulders supported against the headboard or some other solid piece of furniture. She sits between his legs with her ankles wrapped around his neck. Clasping hands and forearms, he pulls her to him and gently pushes her away from him. All the movement is hers. He remains steady.
2. She leans back with her legs wide open, supporting her weight on one or both of her arms. He sits between her legs, with his legs outstretched loosely around her body. He enters her; she wraps her ankles around his neck. Using his legs as leverage, he moves inside her, almost withdrawing his penis on every stroke.

Essential Fusion Tantra Tip:
Take it to the Counter

Have you ever had intercourse with her sitting on the kitchen counter or a washer/dryer and him standing in front? This is a variation on that technique. Here's how it works:

1. *She opens her legs as wide as she comfortably can, while sitting on the counter (or washer/dryer).*

2. *He holds on to her hips, enters her, and thrusts vigorously. Her wide angle facilitates G-spot stimulation and, of course, her hands are free to stimulate her clitoris.*

Top, Position #10;
Bottom, Variation #2

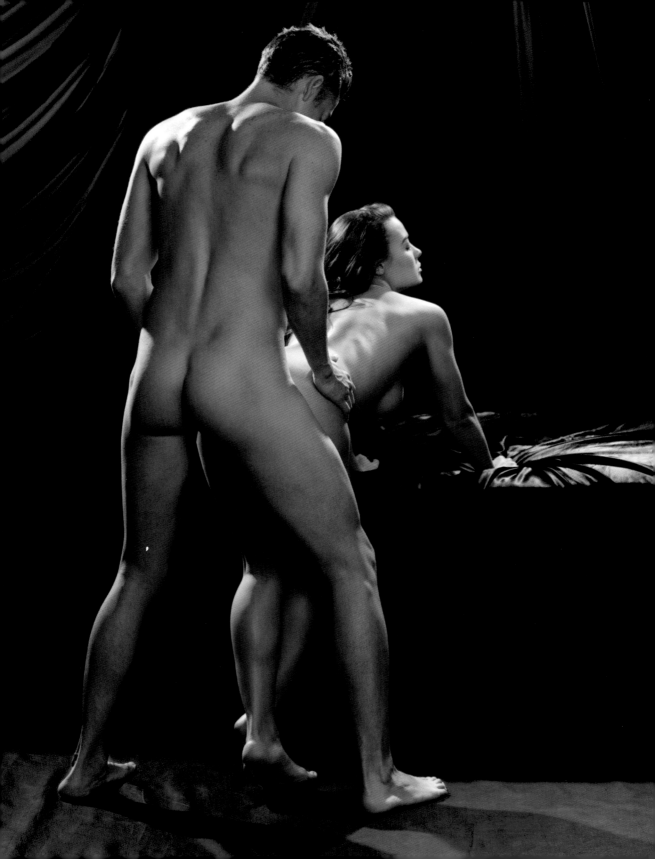

Standing

This position is always associated with hot, urgent, fast sex. The ultimate quickie, the standing position might seem like it is suitable only for young, slender, and fit couples of comparable height. Not true. Almost every book on Tantra—but not this one—has the obligatory photo of standing sex: the man holds the woman, whose legs are wrapped around his waist. Presumably, they have intercourse in this position (which should come with a warning from the American Medical Association about back injuries). Now *that* is difficult. The following two positions are not.

FUSION TANTRA POSITION #11: THE BEND OVER

Adapted from the Kama Sutra position known as "The Cow," the Bend Over employs this simple configuration: they each have both feet on the floor and are facing the same direction.

Following are the benefits of the Bend Over:

- It is well suited to quickies. (And you can both keep your eyes on the door.)

- It can be adapted to couples of differing heights.

- It is exciting.

- It allows direct clitoral stimulation.

The Setup

Here's how the Bend Over works:

1. He stands behind her.
2. She is also standing, with her back toward him. She bends at the waist and leans forward, holding on to a piece of furniture. Or, if she is flexible enough, she can bend all the way forward, fingertips or palms to the floor (as if she were doing the toe-touch exercise).
3. She crosses her ankles as he enters her. That move tightens her vagina.
4. She flexes her PC muscle and the muscles in her buttocks in time to his thrusting.

The Fusion Tantra Difference

Crossing her ankles and flexing her PC muscle intensifies her arousal and helps her reach orgasm sooner.

Variations

1. Standing, she leans forward over a piece of furniture so that she is "lying down" from the waist up. That changes the angle of penetration and gives her greater ability to thrust back against him.
2. Instead of crossing her ankles, she stands with her legs wide apart. Now she has more freedom of movement. (And this position is more comfortable for her if he has a large penis.)

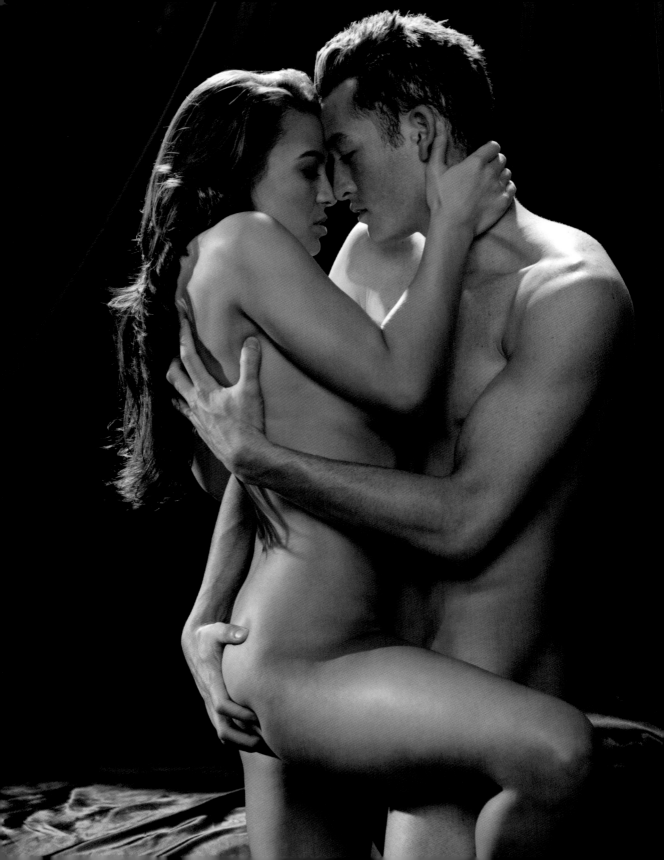

FUSION TANTRA POSITION #12: UP AGAINST THE WALL

Based on the Kama Sutra position "The Supported Congress," this adaptation uses a simple configuration: he stands with his back against the wall for support (or, if he's fit enough, without any wall at all), while she also stands, straddling him with one leg.

Here are some pros to Up Against the Wall:

- It feels dramatic and exciting.

- It works great as a quickie.

The Setup
Here is the rundown for Up Against the Wall:

1. He stands against a wall, with his feet planted comfortably wide apart. If she is several inches shorter than he is, she will need to wear high heels or stand on something, such as a higher step or a sturdy footstool.
2. She spreads her thighs and wraps one leg around his (at the top of his leg level, not waist high).
3. He clasps her thigh or back as he thrusts, with one hand holding her opposite buttock.

The Fusion Tantra Difference
The wall against his back gives him support as he thrusts. By holding her thigh, he makes it easier for her to sustain the standing position, and he gives himself more support. Raising her leg to this level (and not wrapping it around his waist) can make penetration deeper.

Variations
1. In a variation of the Indian Lotus position, each lover wraps one leg around the other. Movement is more restricted. But this is a good position for keeping a semierect penis in place while his excitement builds.
2. She stands against the wall (instead of him standing against it). This gives her more support to wrap her leg around his body.
3. The cheaters' move: She sits almost sideways, with one buttock on a counter or piece of furniture of the right height. Her opposite leg is extended to the floor. Facing her, he enters her. She wraps the unextended leg around his waist. While she is not exactly sitting on the counter, she does have one buttock in place there to support her weight and balance the couple.

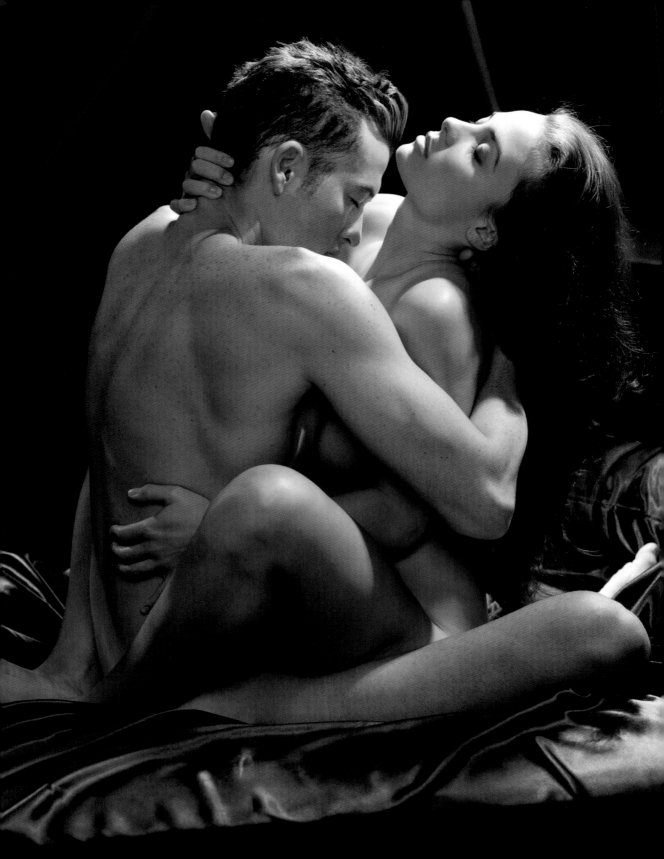

The One Kama Sutra Position *Everyone* Should Know: Yabyum

The classic Yabyum is a variation on a sitting position, but a variation that requires the lovers to be reasonably flexible. Touted as the embodiment of the essential Tantric principles of lovemaking, the Yabyum position encourages her arousal and orgasm, prolongs and delays his orgasm, and promotes intimacy. In fact, it is the ultimate position for delaying orgasm and prolonging intercourse—perfect for a languid Sunday afternoon.

The Setup
Here's how to set up the Yabyum:

1. The couple sits in the center of the bed facing each other.
2. She wraps her legs around his so that she is sitting on his thighs.
3. She places her right hand at the back of his neck; he does the same to her.
4. The couple places their left hands on each other's tailbones. They stroke each other's backs, using upward strokes only. Looking deeply into one another's eyes, they kiss with their eyes open.
5. She puts his semierect penis inside her vagina so it exerts as much indirect pressure as possible on her clitoris and makes G-spot contact. (She can sit on pillows rather than his thighs if necessary to get the angle of penetration right.)
6. They kiss deeply.
7. The couple rocks slowly together while continuing to rub each other's backs and sustaining deep eye contact. They should maintain this position until both reach orgasm.

Variations
By popular demand, I adapted this position to make it easier for the less-than-limber, the knee-injured, pregnant, overweight, and no-longer-as-young-as-we-used-to-be lovers. The changes make it easier, while still giving the same effect.

1. She sits in the center of the bed, on a pillow, facing him. She wraps her legs comfortably around his body. His legs can be splayed straight out or bent at the knees, whatever is more comfortable. She places her right hand at the base of his neck and her left hand at the base of his spine. He should do the same. They caress each other's necks and stroke each other's backs, using upward strokes only. Looking into each other's eyes, they kiss with their eyes open. They should continue kissing and stroking until both are aroused.

   He inserts his penis into her vagina so the shaft exerts as much indirect pressure on her clitoris as possible. They rock together, slowly rubbing each other's backs and kissing deeply with their eyes open for several strokes. Then they open their legs before it gets uncomfortable—generally relaxing the position is what makes it Fusion Tantra.
2. In this variation, he sits on the bed with his legs wide open. She lies back on the bed, facing him, with her body between his legs. She puts her ankles up against his shoulders so he can enter her at a comfortable angle. Her thighs should stay close together, creating a tighter grip on his penis.
3. In this variation, she lies on her back, again between his legs, but with her legs bent at the knees and pulled back against her body until her heels touch (or approximately touch) her thighs. He sits close to her. She pulls him closer until he can comfortably insert his penis.

The Yabyum Position

The Other Kama Sutra Position *Everyone* Should Know: Starfish

The Starfish position goes by several other names, including most often the X, or Scissors. It's also known as *Cuissade*, the French word for thigh. It is perfect for slow, grinding sex. And it doesn't place one lover's weight on the other's body. If you're in the mood for easy, somewhat emotionally detached intercourse, then this is the way to do it. (And many couples would have sex more often if they did occasionally allow themselves to do it in an easy and detached fashion.)

The Setup
Here's how the Starfish works:
1. Both lie on their backs on the bed, the woman lying in a perpendicular position to the man (so if her head is at the head of the bed, his head is at the side).
2. He turns slightly on to his side (toward her) and "scissors" his legs. Imagine an X, with one of his legs under one of hers and his other leg on top of her thigh.
3. Both push their hips together.
4. They adjust their bodies so that penetration will be high, giving her more pressure against her clitoris.
5. He penetrates her.
6. Both clasp arms or hands now, for leverage in movement.
7. The couple rocks back and forth, maintaining a grinding pressure on her clitoris.

Variations
1. Both partners put pillows underneath their back/ sides. This will allow for more vigorous thrusting.
2. She raises her top leg and rests it on his body. He can wrap his arm around this leg. He enters her from beneath her thigh. She uses her thigh to control his thrusting.

Fusion Tantra Quickies

Can you call a quickie "Tantra"? Probably not. But you *can* call a quickie Fusion Tantra if you use the breathing and other techniques to increase arousal.

The quickie is a staple of the modern couple's sex diet. They might only have time for more extended lovemaking once a week—or twice, if they're lucky—but their appetite for arousal and orgasm needs to be sated more often. And, yes, a quickie can work for a woman as well as it does for a man.

To make it happen for her, too:
1. She needs to start on "hot." Some women prefer to slip into the bedroom or bathroom and masturbate until they are aroused. Others incorporate vibrator play into the quickie.
2. She should continue the direct clitoral stimulation (with or without a vibe) during intercourse, if necessary.
3. The couple should adjust positions to ensure she gets as much clitoral stimulation (or G-spot stimulation, if that works for her) as possible.

It's All Worth a Try

Few readers will love every single one of the down-and-dirty Fusion Tantra positions. But how will you know what will work for you and what won't if you don't try them all? I recommend trying each one and, of course, adapting them to your bodies. Without variety, intercourse gets boring. Also, our bodies change over time so the tried-and-true positions might not be so true for us anymore. This is play, not work. If you collapse laughing in a heap while trying one of these positions, that's not a bad thing either.

The Starfish Position

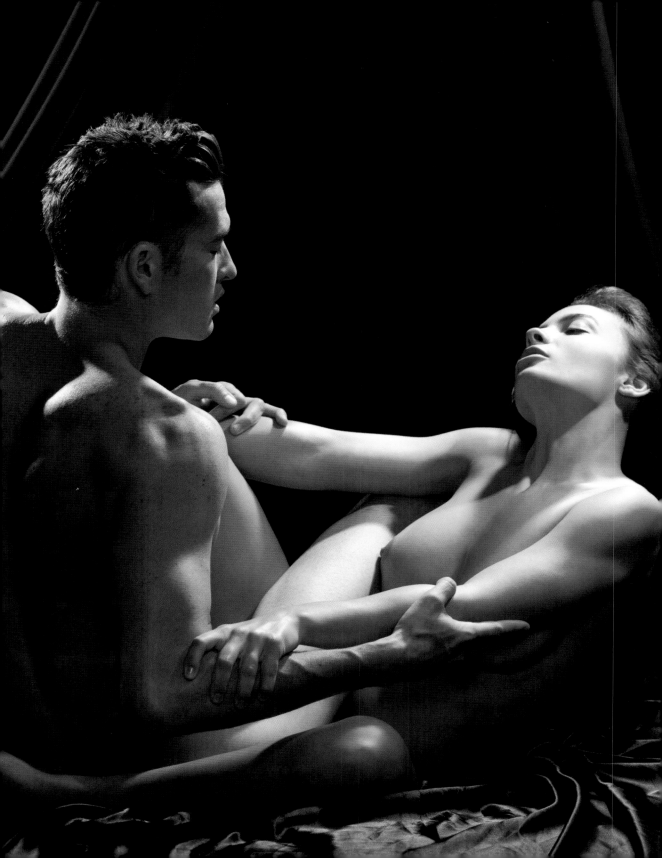

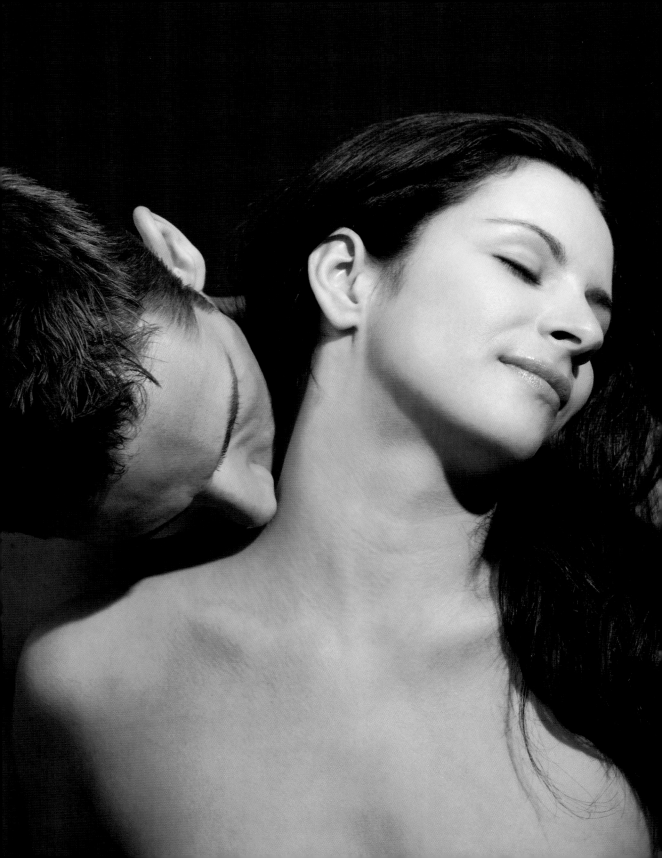

PART 6

Fusion Tantra Wrap-Up

Sex books generally fall into two categories: the books that promise more than they can deliver (or more than you would have the time and energy to enjoy) and the ones that focus obsessively on problems. Scan the shelves in your local bookstore, and you might wonder: what exactly falls between a twenty-four-hour orgasm and a totally dysfunctional woman and her disinterested man?

Beyond those two extremes, when you get right down to it, there is a lot of middle ground, and that is more realistic. In most of our sex lives there are good (even great) times and not so good ones, too. Ups and downs are normal, after all. Fusion Tantra helps you make the most of your sex life. You will have more arousing, orgasmic, and intimate experiences, and you will learn techniques for handling smoothly the little problems that short-circuit a potentially good time and good relationship. Yes, into every sex life an occasional dysfunction falls. Don't worry about that. We can fix it.

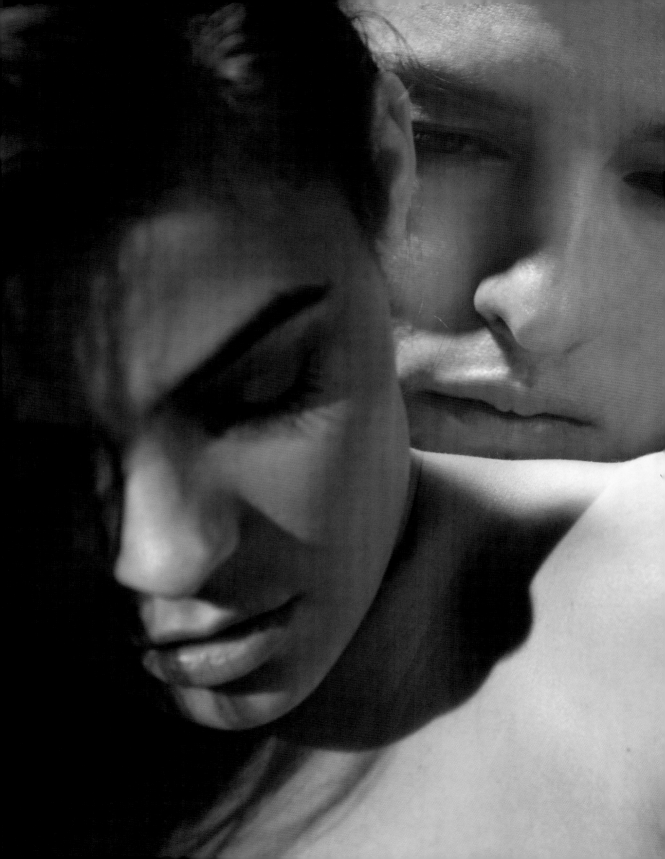

Chapter 15

Sex Complaint?
Fusion Tantra Has the Fix

Thousands of years ago, India's pioneer sexologists realized that sex was problematic unless the speed and intensity of female arousal could be increased and orgasm ensured. At the same time, male arousal had to be prolonged, with ejaculation delayed. That is the basic equation behind the Kama Sutra, Neo-Tantra, and Western sex therapy. The techniques in this section are quick fixes for any problem that gets in the way of that goal.

Common Sex Compliant #1: He Comes Too Fast

First, it's not "over" because he (or she) reaches orgasm. Use hands, mouths, and vibrators to play until both are satisfied.

"He comes too soon" generally means that she doesn't reach orgasm via intercourse alone while he, of course, does. To solve the complaint, give her an orgasm via cunnilingus first. Or, ladies, simply take matters into your own hands and give yourself direct clitoral stimulation during intercourse. Both paths to pleasure are fine—or you can try something new. Read on for more.

❧ FUSION TANTRA TECHNIQUE: **THE SQUEEZE**

Masters and Johnson modeled their famous squeeze technique on a more elegant Taoist version. This squeeze is simpler and equally effective for extending his arousal and delaying his orgasm.

When he feels ejaculation is imminent but not inevitable, he simply withdraws his penis from her vagina. He or she then lightly squeezes the head of his penis for several seconds and they resume intercourse. The squeeze can be repeated two or three times, if necessary.

> "More than one technique for preventing premature ejaculation is derived from Tantra. That's marvelous therapy. But I am not enthralled with the meditation and other aspects of Tantra."
>
> —SUE JOHANSON,
> Canadian sex expert

❦ FUSION TANTRA TECHNIQUE: **ALTERNATING STIMULI OR STOP/START**

Another Western sex therapy classic, this one has its roots in both Taoist and Tantra traditions that encourage prolonged male arousal. By alternating intercourse with other forms of lovemaking, most men can "last" longer.

The steps are simple: He stops thrusting when he is highly aroused, but not near orgasm, and continues arousing her, manually or orally or with a vibe. (She does not touch his erection.) He resumes intercourse when arousal subsides, before losing his erection.

He can repeat this process several times during lovemaking, bringing her to more than one orgasm manually or orally or with a vibe.

❦ FUSION TANTRA TECHNIQUE: **SHE TAKES OVER**

Women enjoy penetration as much as men do. Sometimes she wants the thrusting to last longer. And the techniques for delaying his orgasm also interrupt the thrusting. What to do? Take charge. Tease and taunt him.

The female superior position is the best one for her to control the thrusting, and it gives her the maximum clitoral stimulation from intercourse while reducing the intense head of the penis friction that gives him an orgasm. Here's how to do it:

1. She lowers herself on to *only the head* of his penis and pulls back repeatedly. (The teasing slows down his arousal while sustaining his erection.)

2. She plays with her clitoris while she's playing that game with him. (Use fingers or a small vibe.)

3. She holds his hands over his head and runs her tongue all over his body while grinding her clitoris into his pubic bone.

4. She continues to deprive him of sustained friction on the head of his penis until she is near orgasm. Then she mounts him.

Common Sex Complaint #2: She Takes Too Long to Come (or She Can't Reach Orgasm During Intercourse)

When people ask me what I have found most surprising in twenty-five years of studying, researching, interviewing, and writing about sex, I always reply: that women still ask, "How can I come during intercourse?" meaning *without touching myself*.

Men like to think that they "give" us orgasms, but mostly they do not. Even in cunnilingus, she leads him by thrusting her clitoris against his mouth and tongue. By manipulating intercourse positions to get the stimulation we need, by strengthening and using our PC muscle, by using our hands, vibes, or the Orgasm Loop, we can take what we need for ourselves. That women have traditionally not done so says more about cultural conditioning—across cultures—than it does about anatomy and physiology. *You* can reach orgasm whenever you want by:

- Increasing PC strength and using that muscle during intercourse.

- Incorporating breathing, PC techniques, and energy focus into foreplay.

- Using the Orgasm Loop.

- Adding vibe play to sex.

- Asking him to stimulate your clitoris during intercourse.

Take charge of your orgasm and you are free to enjoy all the wonderful things he is doing to your body. Wait for him to "give" you an orgasm and you miss a lot of the sensations because you are tense waiting for "it" to happen. The essence of traditional Tantric sex teachings (and the Kama Sutra) was that he is responsible for your pleasure and should delay, even sacrifice, his own pleasure to ensure yours. The essence of Fusion Tantra is that we as women need to take responsibility for our own orgasms so that we can fully surrender to the joys of sex.

Common Sex Complaint #3: The Sex Is Boring

That complaint propelled your mama into Neo-Tantra! Lucky for you though, there are quick fixes in every section of this book for this garden-variety sex problem that afflicts all of us at one time or another—and you don't have to clear your chakras first. Try out any of the intercourse positions and variations in chapter 14 and you'll surely cure your boredom in no time.

Common Sex Complaint #4: I've Lost the Desire (or I Don't Think I Love Him Anymore Because I Don't Desire Him)

I wrote about the Desire Curve (created with Nan Wise) in my book *The Sex Bible for Women*. A simple and elegant theory, the Desire Curve maps out the desire patterns in relationships and explains how they work. What we perceive as loss of desire is typically loss of *spontaneous* desire—the heady feeling of wanting sex with a lover when you see or even think about him (or her).

After eighteen months to three years in a new relationship, that spontaneous desire goes away. In its place is *receptive* desire. If you become aroused when your lover kisses, touches, or strokes you, then you have receptive desire. The techniques in Fusion Tantra help you get in touch with that receptive desire.

How? By using these techniques:

- Energizing your whole body to make you feel more sexually alive and more desirous of sex.

- Intensifying your awareness of arousal (which women often ignore).

- Giving yourself greater control over your orgasms; the more orgasmic you are, the more you will desire sex.

- Creating greater intimacy between you and your lover, making sex more frequent. The more sex you have, the more in touch you are with your own desire—and the more sex you want to have.

Common Sex Complaint #5: I Just Want the Sex to End!

An astonishing percentage of women—older, younger, richer, poorer, educated, and less so—fake orgasms. Some surveys and studies say as many as 85 percent of all women have faked (or routinely fake) orgasms. And the number one reason for faking: "I just wanted the sex to end."

Why would a woman want the sex to end? Here are some possibilities:

- She never became fully aroused and was too tired, stressed, or out of sync to get there.
- He wanted sex badly and she submitted to please him.
- Something short-circuited her arousal and then she just wanted to stop.
- She came first and lost interest before he came. (Some women fake the "second," or intercourse, orgasm.)

He might not be able make her come whenever he wants, but she can almost always make him come, especially if she has a strong PC muscle and knows her way around a male perineum. The boys can't help it. The trajectory of male arousal to orgasm is more straightforward than that of women. Women must think of that trajectory as a line that they can shorten or lengthen, and then do that sometimes just because they can.

FUSION TANTRA TECHNIQUE: MAKE HIM COME WITH THE G-SPOT ORGASM

A G-spot orgasm is powerful, sending vibrations throughout his body. And you can do this any time you want, either to end the sex or because you enjoy giving him intense pleasure.

Stroke his perineum during fellatio or while you are giving him a hand job. Or insert a finger into his anus. If he is responsive, come back there later; if not, skip this section. Once you know that he (like most men) is amenable to the G-spot stroke:

- Excite him to the point of orgasm via oral and manual stimulation to his penis using techniques on pages 84-87.
- Stop the stimulation abruptly, when he's really getting into it. He will beg for more; and you will give it to him.

- Hold his thighs apart when you notice him writhing in ecstasy, and lower your mouth to his perineum.

- Flick your tongue rapidly back and forth across that area.

- Press your thumb lightly against his perineum—gauging the pressure by his response—as you continue flicking your tongue.

- If he's into anal play, you can insert a well-lubed finger into his anus and stroke the perineum from inside.

❧ FUSION TANTRA TECHNIQUE:
MAKE HIM COME WITH THE ROUGH TOUCH

Take a page from the Kama Sutra, specifically one of those pages about pinching, biting, and slapping—activities heartily endorsed in the good book.

- Pinch or bite his nipple during intercourse, when he is highly aroused but not yet at the point of inevitability.

- Create a pause in the coital dynamics by clenching your PC and squeezing his penis tightly.

- Grab his buttocks if you can reach them.

- Use your PC muscle to pull him in deeper. Make eye contact with him at the same time.

- Pinch or bite his nipple again. He will come.

Patterns Were Meant to Be Broken

Most sex "problems" aren't major issues. Sometimes the sex doesn't seem to be working because we're tired, stressed, bored, or emotionally disconnected from our partners. An occasional lackluster lovemaking session is no big deal, but you don't want that to become the pattern of your sex life. That's why every lover needs these techniques. Remember the basics: increase and intensify her arousal and orgasm, prolong his arousal, and delay his orgasm.

Trust me on this: It's not the relationship that's wrong; it's the sex. You will like each other a lot better if the sex is good.

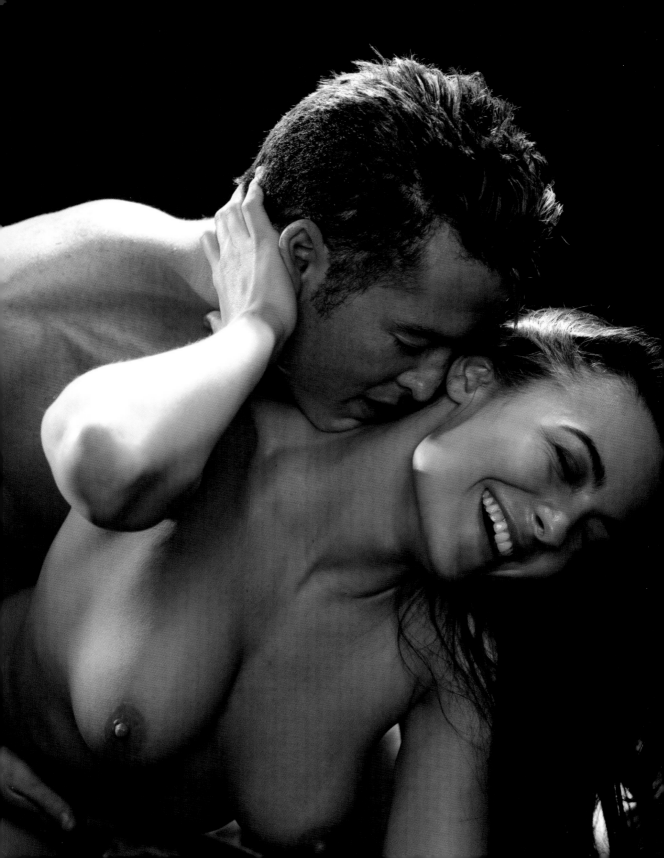

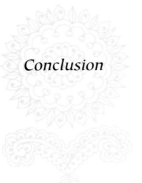

Conclusion

The Take-Away Lessons of Fusion Tantra

I hope this book has taught you how to:

- Add erotic breathing and breath control to your sex life.

- Do your Kegel exercises and strengthen the PC muscle.

- Feel your sexual energy—and move it around at will.

- Be creative with intercourse positions and make them work to suit your bodies.

- Let her take charge of her orgasms (and even sometimes his).

- Stay in the sexual moment.

Get out of your "busy talk" head and into your sexual body. It's all good from there. I would never claim to be your orgasm messenger from God, knowing all of the answers about everything all of the time. Just think of me as your Auntie Mame of Sex, telling you in a (more or less) respectful way that Mama had this Tantra sex thing all wrong. But there's good news! I found the naughty bits just for you.

Sex should be at least a little naughty to be fun. Your mama's Tantra wasn't a down-and-dirty game. Ever. The pursuit of soul-touching intimacy might be a higher calling, but like the convent, it has never called to me.

Whether or not it calls to you, you can use the techniques in this book to make your sex life hotter and your love connection more intimate. Fusion Tantra is for the busy, the tired and stressed, the happily coupled and the happily single, anyone in need of a quick sex fix. You don't have to commit a lot of time to learning the techniques. There is no "woo woo" here. No pretensions. This is simple and sexy—just like you wish your sex life could be.

Acknowledgments

Who ever accomplishes anything without the support of many people?

First, thank you to my agent, Richard Curtis.

A big thanks to the wonderful Quiver team, the people who make these beautiful books: Will Kiester, publisher; Jill Alexander, senior editor; Rosalind Wanke, creative director; Amanda Waddell, project editor; Karen Levy, copyeditor; and the brilliant design group.

And special thanks to Andrea Mattei, super-smart and witty developmental editor who makes me look good.

Thanks also to the beautiful models featured in this book.

Everybody has an emotional support team, and I am grateful to mine. My dearest longtime friends: Carolyn Males, Michael and Barb Hasamear, Alex Zola, and Joe Rinaldi.

My daughter-in-law, Tamm, who gave us the incomparable Marcella and her new twin brothers, Alex and Evan. They are just starting to smile as I wrap up this book.

Nan Wise, new friend, colleague, and collaborator; her wonderful husband, John; and their delightful (and wise beyond her years) daughter, Julia.

My Harlem friends in the 'hood: Elizabeth and Reggie, Val Bradley, Kathryn Williams, and everyone at St. Nick's Pub and at Native restaurant.

The great researchers who have taught and inspired me: Dr. Eileen Palace, Dr. Barry Komisaruk, Dr. Gina Ogden, the late sexologist Marc Meshorer, and Dr. Annie Sprinkle.

And Barbara Carrellas, whose Urban Tantra encouraged me to explore my own vision of Fusion Tantra.

About the Author

SUSAN CRAIN BAKOS is an internationally recognized sex authority and author of twelve books, including *The Sex Bible: The Complete Guide to Sexual Love* and *The Orgasm Loop*. She has been writing about sex for more than two decades, with her work appearing in such magazines as *Redbook*, *Cosmopolitan*, *Men's Health*, and *Penthouse*.

A former contributing editor and columnist at *Penthouse Forum*, Susan has worked with such legends as Dr. Ruth Westheimer and Helen Gurley Brown and has interviewed thousands of men and women about their sex lives. She has also appeared on *Oprah*, *Good Morning America*, and numerous other television and radio shows. She lives in New York City and holds steadfast to the belief that every woman should own a wardrobe of vibrators and have at least one orgasm a day. Check out her blog at sexyprime.typepad.com.